Testosterone

A Clinical Review

Mark W DelBello MD FACP CDE

© 2017 Mark W DelBello MD FACP CDE
All rights reserved.

ISBN: 1545586179
ISBN 13: 9781545586174
Library of Congress Control Number: 2017906676
CreateSpace Independent Publishing Platform
North Charleston, South Carolina

Table of Contents

Preface	v
Introduction	vii
Overview	1
Muscle Mass	11
More Supportive Evidence for Testosterone	16
Testosterone and Surgical Outcomes	50
Testosterone and Prostate	62
Levels/logistics of testosterone	71
Growth Hormone	84
Muscle Beach	105
Sarcopenia (poverty of the flesh)	128
Exercise	152
Inflammation and the gut	170
Women and testosterone	174
Evidence not supporting testosterone	186
Conclusion	199
References	201

Preface

THIS IS A REFERENCE BOOK to help people understand and potentially appreciate testosterone. Testosterone usage has been controversial in the past and continues to be. This book tries to answer some questions about what it does and does not do along with potential benefits and pitfalls with it. The book is really for medical students, physicians, nurses, physician assistants, nurse practitioners, and research oriented people. A lay person will understand parts but may find it too scientific, clinical and complicated.

The articles have been chosen for their merit and all credit belongs to the authors of them. I have shortened the length of most for reading convenience. The words are the authors and not mine. The ideas belong to the authors and they deserve all the credit. My role was to bring gifted physicians and researchers together in a relatively short book to bring these ideas under one roof. It is also important to realize that minorities have been mostly left out of the research, and this needs to change to provide a more complete and accurate picture.

Introduction

UNTIL RECENTLY, IT WAS THOUGHT that testosterone deficiency in middle-aged men and older men mainly affected the quality of life, but it was unlikely to affect morbidity or mortality. However, population-based studies indicate that testosterone deficiency predicts future development of type 2 diabetes, metabolic syndrome, cardiovascular events, mobility limitation, frailty, and mortality. (Cunningham & Toma, 2011) (Ding, Song, Malik, & Liu, 2006) (Laaksonen, et al., 2004) (Krasnoff, et al., 2010) (Hyde, et al., 2010) (Laughlin, Barrett-Connor, & Bergstrom, 2008) (Khaw, et al., 2007) (Menke, et al., 2010) (Maggio, et al., 2007). Modest reductions in skeletal muscle mass with aging do not cause functional impairment and disability: however, when skeletal muscle mass relative to body weight is 30% below the mean of young adults, an increase risk of functional impairment and disability is found. The development of sarcopenia (muscle loss) in the elderly is not the result of one single change occurring during aging but is a consequence of multisystem change. If the decline in physical function in the frail elderly can be sufficiently reversed, then the gains in muscle mass and strength may be retained by improved functional capacity, breaking the downward cycle of ever increasing weakness and debility (Bauman, La Fountaine, Cirnigliaro, Kirshblum, & Spungen, 2015). The age-related decline in testosterone levels is caused by defects at all levels of the hypothalamic-pituitary-testicular axis, and the trajectory of decline is affected by BMI, weight gain, comorbid conditions, medications and genetic factors. By combining symptoms, total testosterone levels and sometimes Luteinizing Hormone (LH) levels, the accuracy of the diagnosis of hypogonadism may improve (Spitzer, Huang, Basaria, Travison, & Bhasin, 2013). An essential question is whether this decrease in the testosterone concentration is physiologic, perhaps conveying a benefit, or pathologic, causing harm. This book should provide clarity.

Overview

TESTOSTERONE IS THE PRINCIPAL SECRETED androgen in men. An androgen is a sex hormone that promotes the development and maintenance of the male sex characteristics. Androgens have both androgenic effects (masculinizing effects- development of male sex characteristics, including hair growth) and anabolic effects (increase in skeletal muscle mass and strength).

Testosterone increases skeletal muscle mass by inducing the hypertrophy of both type 1 and type 2 muscle fibers. Testosterone does not change the absolute number or the relative proportion of type 1 and 2 fibers. It does increase the number of muscle progenitor cells (satellite cells), which contribute to muscle fiber hypertrophy. Testosterone increases maximal voluntary strength and leg power. It promotes mitochondrial biogenesis and increases net oxygen delivery to the tissues by increasing red cell mass and tissue capillarity. Testosterone increases levels of 2,3 biphosphoglycerate, which shifts the oxygen-hemoglobin curve to the left, thereby facilitating oxygen unloading from oxyhemoglobin. The observation that testosterone improves neuromuscular transmission and upregulates acetylcholinesterase expression in the frog hind limb model have led to speculation that testosterone may reduce reaction time, which may contribute to improved performance in sprint events or in sports requiring a high level of hand-eye coordination, such as baseball. The baseball players Bobby Bonds and Alex Rodriguez are good examples.

General theory states that the decline in testosterone level occurs either simply in some older men or the decline is a result of accumulation of comorbidities such as obesity, heart disease, diabetes, etc. Theses 2 subsets of men with low T predominate the situation. The average decline in T levels with aging is 1-2% per year. T levels, after peaking in the second and third decade of life decline gradually with advancing age without a clear inflection point or andro-pause. T decreases very gradually with time which is much different than women and estrogen. About 30% of men with a mildly low T level will have a normal level on repeat testing. By the 8th decade, 30% of men had total T levels in the hypogonadal range and 50% had low free T values. Acute illness, excessive exercise, and opiates can decrease T levels. Some endocrine experts think treating low T should occur at 300 ng/dl and some feel it should be less than 200 ng/dl. The conventional definition for hypogonadism is statistical (values more than 2 standard deviations below the mean), rather than functional. **It would clearly be better to define the lower limit of normal for a hormone as: the blood level at which metabolic and/or clinical sequelae of hormone deficiency begin to appear, or the level at which definite benefits can be demonstrated for hormone supplementation.**

In patients with documented coronary artery disease, testosterone deficiency is common and impacts negatively on survival. Excess mortality was noted in a study of androgen-deficient men compared with a control group of normal men. The only parameters found to influence time to all-cause and vascular mortality were the presence of left ventricular dysfunction, ASA therapy, B- blocker therapy, and low T level in the study.

OVERVIEW

There is no other tissue that declines more dramatically with aging than skeletal muscle. This decline starts in the third decade of life and is associated with an even more striking decline of muscle strength and power, as has been shown in both longitudinal and cross-sectional studies (Giannoulis, Martin, Nair, Umpleby, & Sonksen, 2012). **Muscle mass is controlled by the diurnal balance between muscle protein synthesis and protein breakdown. Testosterone regulates many physiological processes and each process may have different dose-response relationships.** Organ systems respond differently to testosterone levels. For example, libido, erectile dysfunction and mood respond to levels more in the low normal range whereas skeletal muscle responds to higher levels in a dose dependent manner. Androgen deficiency and erectile dysfunction, despite the impression that they are closely related, really are two distinct syndromes that are independently distributed in men. By prioritizing the goals of T therapy, we can better choose desired levels making it potentially safer to use.

Regular resistance training three times per week is the best way to maintain muscle mass but testosterone therapy may be an acceptable lesser way for people unable to exercise due to co-morbidities. Exercise is the most powerful physiological stimulus for Growth Hormone secretion which decreases also with aging. Heavy resistance exercise has not shown to elicit the same magnitude of hormonal responses (i.e. muscle mass, protein synthesis) in younger men (30 years old) versus older men (62 years old). The hypertrophic response of muscle to training in older men is blunted when compared with younger counterparts, and this has been attributed to the deficient anabolic hormone profile and locally expressed milieu (Giannoulis, Martin, Nair, Umpleby, & Sonksen, 2012).

TESTOSTERONE — A CLINICAL REVIEW

Testosterone use has been under a cloud of fear that it may cause more harm than benefit. Double-blind placebo-controlled trials looking at hard end points such as cardiovascular events, and soft end points such as quality of life require studies of a duration and study size so large that realistically it probably will not happen. Treatment of testosterone deficiency due to classical diseases affecting the hypothalamus, pituitary, and/or testes has been accepted for decades, although there were no multi-center trials. **The true debate revolves whether treating a low testosterone level is a modifiable risk factor that can result in improved health, longevity and shorter duration of chronic illness. The debate is complicated further because testosterone is metabolized by 5-alpha-reductase into dihydrotestosterone (DHT), which competes for the androgen receptor, and is also metabolized by aromatase into estradiol, which competes for the estrogen receptor.** To expect hormone replacement therapy to improve an outcome in a statistical manner over a short study time that may have required years or decades to develop might be expecting too much. Most organ systems, hormones and drugs work best within a range. Levels above and below those ranges may not be beneficial or may promote increased morbidity and mortality. Most medicines have therapeutic windows and testosterone is no exception. Sulfonylurea agents and warfarin account for nearly half of adverse drug events leading to the emergent hospitalization of elderly and we still use these products frequently. Using the erythrocytosis side effect of testosterone can be used to our advantage to lessen the need for transfusions for surgery. Androgen therapy may reduce the risk of re-hospitalization in older men with testosterone deficiency and this intervention potentially holds broad clinical and public health relevance. It's important to know that testosterone treatment will suppress gonadotropins and spermatogenesis. It is not appropriate for treatment of testosterone-deficient men who desire to father a child in the future.

Epidemiological studies report increased mortality in men with low testosterone. T replacement in the short term reduces waist circumference, cholesterol and circulating pro-inflammatory cytokines and improves insulin sensitivity and glycemic control in diabetics. Testosterone also has beneficial effects on cardiac ischemia, angina, and congestive heart failure. Studies on androgen ablation therapy are very instructive regarding quality of life and cardiac risk. Atherosclerosis is now recognized as an inflammatory disease, with evidence of inflammatory cells at the level of the plaque and in the circulation. The hypothalamic-pituitary-testicular axis is suppressed by inflammatory cytokines such as interleukin-1, interleukin-6, and TNF-alpha. It can therefore be postulated that any disease associated with an inflammatory state promotes T deficiency, and low T could be considered a biomarker of illness (Jones, 2010).

A different philosophy may be required to appreciate the benefits of some hormone replacement therapy. What is physiologically relevant may not be statistically significant in time limited studies using physiological and supra-physiological drug doses? For example, a 10% loss of bone mass in the vertebrae can double the risk of vertebral fractures, and similarly, a 10% loss of bone mass in the hip can result in a 2.5 times greater risk of hip fracture (Klotzbuecher, Ross, Landsman, Abbott, & Berger, 2000). People fracture bones because their reserve both in muscle strength and bone strength decrease to a dangerous level that has no margin of error. 10% may not seem statistically significant but it may be the difference between independent living and a nursing home to a person living on the edge with little functional reserve. Think of Olympic athletes and how the smallest of margins decide between an Olympic gold versus 4th place.

Non-prescription "Over-the-counter testosterone boosters and products may carry hidden dangers. There's not a lot of scientific evidence for any supplement that claims to boost or promote testosterone. These products have been around forever. A man who thinks he's short on testosterone shouldn't be looking in a health food store for answers. He needs to go to a doctor to get checked out" (Woolston, 2011).

Many people are treated with testosterone without measuring a level. That would be like treating women for "presumed hypothyroidism" without adequate bloodwork, commencing with maximal dose thyroxine and then concluding that thyroid replacement was highly dangerous (Hackett G. , 2016). Medicines are not harmless choices. Cause and effect relationships are hard to prove but that should not discourage us from using data to help advance the treatment of many medical conditions. Difficult questions require large numbers of participants over a long duration of time and many times the studies will never be done for practical or financial reasons. I have chosen articles regarding testosterone to provide fair balance. Many articles express similar ideas not by my biased selection but to emphasize state of the art thinking. Several recurring principles are repeated in multiple studies providing multiple avenues of evidence. Education and truth are always powerful tools. A criticism of my research is that most studies do not involve minorities so the picture is not complete. My personal belief is testosterone therapy will become the standard of care in preoperative protocols, hospital protocols and that its administration will be done in a more responsible professional manner.

OVERVIEW

The following study shows how testosterone may be the standard of care in the future:

Effects of testosterone supplementation on clinical and rehabilitative outcomes in older men undergoing on-pump CABG

When older men with low ejection fractions undergo cardiac revascularization with extracorporeal circulation, there is a profound decline in anabolic hormones, including testosterone. After surgery testosterone concentration frequently declines to less than 200 ng/dl, a situation suggestive of overt hypogonadism. Since men with low testosterone levels have a high probability of developing mobility limitations, we considered this a rationale for the perioperative use of testosterone treatment in older men undergoing cardiac revascularization surgery. Men with low testosterone levels have a 57% probability of developing mobility limitations, and a 68% probability of worsening these limitations over the next 4-8 years compared with men with normal free testosterone levels. Epidemiological studies suggest an opportunity for preoperative testosterone treatment to attenuate the catabolic postoperative profile and to potentially improve postoperative outcomes. With attenuation of the catabolic state, an improvement of physical function is also predicted.

Indexes of functional recovery will be measured by the Short Physical Performance Battery (3 separate measures of lower extremity function). The three tests include walking speed, ability to stand 5 times from a chair (arms crossed), and ability to maintain balance in side-to-side, semi-tandem and full-tandem positions. A 6-minute walk test will be measured.

The secondary aim of this study is to test the effects of testosterone treatment for 12 weeks on anabolic and catabolic hormones, inflammatory markers, and body composition as possible mediators of the relationship between testosterone and physical outcomes. Ideally, treatment will increase anabolic hormones, reduce systemic markers of inflammation, improve mood and quality of life, decrease the number of transfusions and shorten rehabilitation period. Currently, it is not known whether the testosterone decline observed after cardiac surgery is only a physiological and compensatory response to surgical stress or whether this hormonal change has a key role in the development of anemia, inflammation and other adverse outcomes in the postoperative period. (Maggio, et al., 2012)

Another ongoing study evaluates if testosterone can help spinal cord injury patients decrease their tendency to develop an unfavorable metabolic profile. **Effects of Testosterone and Evoked Resistance Exercise after Spinal Cord Injury (TEREX-SCI): study protocol for a randomized controlled trial**

Individuals with spinal cord injury (SCI) are at a lifelong risk of obesity and chronic metabolic disorders including insulin resistance and dyslipidemia. Within a few weeks of injury, there is a significant decline in whole body fat-free mass, particularly lower extremity skeletal muscle mass, and subsequent increase in fat mass (FM). This is accompanied by a decrease in anabolic hormones including testosterone. There are approximately 11,000-12,000 new cases of spinal cord injury in the USA annually with an overall prevalence of 250,000-400,000. Chronic SCI, defined as 1 year postinjury, is associated with dramatic skeletal muscle atrophy, increase of fat mass6-8 and decrease of fat-free mass (6,7). Previous studies reveal that 60% of individuals with SCI in the USA are either overweight or obese. More than 50% of individuals with SCI are glucose intolerant, while one of five is diabetic (2,9-11,21). Previous studies have shown that 60% of men with SCI have low T and that testosterone replacement therapy increases IGF-1 (i.e. GH) in men. 26 individuals with chronic, motor complete SCI between 18 and 50 years old were randomly assigned to a RT (resistance training) and TRT (testosterone replacement therapy) (n=13) or a TRT group (n=13) for 16 weeks. The TRT was provided via transdermal testosterone patches. Electrically evoked RT using neuromuscular electrical stimulation and ankle weights has been shown to be effective in inducing muscle hypertrophy in individuals with chronic SCI. A previous study showed a 40% increase in skeletal muscle size and improved glucose tolerance after 12 weeks of training. Results are not present yet. (Gorgey, et al., 2017)

Testosterone Concentrations in Diabetic and Nondiabetic Obese Men

Free testosterone concentrations of 1,849 men (1,451 nondiabetic and 398 diabetic) in the Hypogonadism in Males (HIM) study were analyzed. The HIM study was a U.S based cross-sectional study designed to define the prevalence of hypogonadism in men aged > 45 years.

Subnormal free T concentrations

	Non-Diabetic	Diabetic
LEAN	26%	44%
Overweight	29%	44%
Obese	40%	50%

The prevalence of a low testosterone level in men greater than 45 years old with diabetics is at least 44% and the prevalence without diabetes is over 25%.

It is significant clinically that the prevalence of hypogonadotropic hypogonadism is greater than 50% in patients with type 2 diabetes aged between 18 and 35 years. Both obesity and diabetes appear to exert independent effects on the prevalence of low free testosterone concentrations in addition to age. (Dhindsa, et al., 2010)

Muscle Mass

MAINTAINING MUSCLE MASS IS ONE of the key points in this book and is also one of the best ways to avoid unhealthy weight. When we lose muscle mass we increase our chances of becoming overweight or obese. Muscle mass essentially determines resting energy expenditure (metabolism) and this declines at about 35 years old. **Testosterone levels decrease both in men and women with age but this cannot be the simple answer. The explanation is multifactorial since many hormone levels decrease with age along with the slow degeneration of most organ systems.**

Trained muscle consumes 9 kcals/lb./day and untrained muscle consumes 5-6 kcals/lb./day. If one eats the same amount every year and does not increase energy expenditure either through work or exercise they will gain weight each year typically starting at 35 years-old. Exercise is really one of the wonders of the world. Six pounds of muscle are lost per decade, metabolic rate decreases 3% per decade, and 16 pounds of fat are gained per decade.

Over the last three years I have noticed how patients absolutely abhor physical activity and exercise. Many people do not grow up with exercise playing a part of their lives and now it's like learning a foreign language. Age does not matter either, I could be talking to a first-year college student or a 45-year-old bank executive. I tell people that walking is the best physical activity and is essential for any quality of life. When people stop walking they turn to rust and become sarcopenic. Sarcopenia is probably the biggest reason for falls as we age. It is a synonym for frailty or adult failure to thrive. It is defined as having decreased upper extremity muscle mass that is two or more standard deviations below a healthy adult 18-40 years old along a low walking speed below 1.8 mph in a 4-minute walking test. Normal walking speed is 3.1 mph. A tortoise does not beat the rabbit if he falls all the time.

A few muscle mass statistics are below;
1. 6-8% muscle mass loss before 50 years.
2. 8-10% muscle mass loss after 50 years and before 70 years.
3. 15% loss after 70 years and continues every decade. About 14% of people 65-75 years old require help in basic ADLs, a proportion that increases to 45% in people over 85.
4. Muscle mass loss is greater in men as compared to women.
   Basic principles for Testosterone
5. T circulates in the body bound to either SHBG (sex hormone binding globulin), albumin or corticosteroid binding globulin (CBG), or in an unbound form (free).
6. SHBG-bound T is tightly bound and unavailable to cells- 44%
7. Albumin-bound T is weakly bound and dissociates easily- 50%
8. CBG-bound T is weakly bound and dissociates rapidly- 4%

9. Free T represents only 2-3% of the total T.
10. "bioavailable T" refers to the sum of the CBG-bound (4%), albumin-bound (50%) and free T (2-3%) and represents the T fraction that is available to cells-56%.

Fundamental Concepts Regarding Testosterone Deficiency and Treatment. International Expert Consensus Resolutions.

To address widespread concerns regarding the medical condition of testosterone (T) deficiency (TD) (male hypogonadism) and its treatment with T therapy, an international expert consensus conference was convened in Prague, Czech Republic, on October 1, 2015. Experts included a broad range of medical specialties including urology, endocrinology, diabetology, internal medicine, and basic science research. A representative from the European Medicines Agency participated in a nonvoting capacity. Nine resolutions were debated, with unanimous approval:

(1) TD is a well-established, clinically significant medical condition that negatively affects male sexuality, reproduction, general health, and quality of life;
(2) symptoms and signs of TD occur because of low levels of T and may benefit from treatment regardless of whether there is an identified underlying etiology; Symptoms and signs occur at different T levels. Erectile dysfunction becomes more common below 233 ng/dl. Depression and type 2 diabetes more common below 288 ng/dl. increased visceral fat below 346 ng/dl and vigor/strength below 433 ng/dl

(3) TD is a global public health concern; In a U.S. study, only about 12% received T therapy despite adequate access to medical care.

(4) T therapy for men with TD is effective, rational, and evidence based.

(5) There is no T concentration threshold that reliably distinguishes those who will respond to treatment from those who will not; Free T may better reflect the clinical androgen status of some patients

(6) there is no scientific basis for any age-specific recommendations against the use of T therapy in men; In light of increased life expectancy, we find no justification to recommend restricting T therapy based on age. The results of the Testosterone Trials, performed in men aged 65 years and older, confirm significant benefits of T therapy in older men and had fewer hospitalizations.

(7) the evidence does not support increased risks of cardiovascular events with T therapy; There has been substantial evidence accumulated over more than 2 decades, indicating that low T concentrations are associated with increased CV risks and that higher T concentrations appear cardioprotective.

(8) the evidence does not support increased risk of prostate cancer with T therapy; A clinical guideline recommendation from the European Association of Urology states that T therapy may be considered after successful treatment of prostate cancer.

(9) the evidence supports a major research initiative to explore possible benefits of T therapy for cardiometabolic disease, including diabetes. Mortality rates are

reduced by half in men with TD who received T therapy compared with untreated men in observational studies. Among men who received T therapy, those with normalized T levels had a reduced rate of CV events/mortality vs men with persistently low T.

These resolutions may be considered points of agreement by a broad range of experts based on the best available scientific evidence (Morgentaler, et al., 2016).

More Supportive Evidence for Testosterone

Bits of information

- It has been well established that men with DM2 have lower T levels compared with nondiabetic men. This association was first reported by 2 investigators in 1978 and since then has been confirmed by greater than 20 additional studies.
- Hemoglobin levels in prepubertal boys and girls are similar but increase in boys after age 13 years mirroring changes in T levels. These data suggest that T contributes to the 1-2 g/dl difference between adult men and women.
- Older persons with low T levels tend to have lower hemoglobin levels, more likely to have anemia, and have a higher risk of developing anemia over a three- year follow-up period.
- A low T level increase the susceptibility to anemia but may not be a sufficient causal factor for anemia, probably because anemia in older persons is multifactorial.
- The erythrocytosis activity of androgens is relatively erythropoietin independent. Before erythropoietic agent stimulants (EAS) were used to treat anemia of renal failure, testosterone was given routinely to increase hemoglobin levels in dialysis patients.

MORE SUPPORTIVE EVIDENCE FOR TESTOSTERONE

- Anemia promotes an increased risk of falls, fractures, cognitive impairment, sarcopenia, mortality and decreased physical ability. Anemic men older than 85 years had more than twice the risk of death than men without anemia.
- Men with Klinefelter syndrome (chronic hypogonadism) have an increased incidence of DM. The prevalence of the metabolic syndrome in adult patients with Klinefelter syndrome can be as high as 44%, compared with 10% in normal controls. (i.e. hypogonadism promotes insulin resistance). The association between the two is not coincidental. Nearly one-third of men with DM have low T levels.
- The American Heart Association published a science advisory paper that notes a link between androgen deprivation therapy for prostate cancer and possible increased cardiovascular risk.
- Antagonists to T (GnRH agonists)-marked loss of bone mineral density, increase in fat mass, loss of muscle mass/strength, hot flashes, decrease libido. Side effects when treating prostate cancer.
- In postmenopausal women, studies show that conventional estrogen replacement has substantial adverse effects: trials of ultralow estrogen replacement have demonstrated beneficial effects. The same idea is not true with testosterone
- A recent meta-analysis of available random controlled trials (29 studies, 1930 patients) indicate that T therapy significantly improves erectile function, sexual-related erections, and sexual desire. The Testosterone Trials confirmed significant benefits of T therapy vs placebo for erections, libido, and sexual activity. In a separate meta-analysis (59 RCTs, 5078 patients), T therapy was found to significantly

reduce fat mass and increase muscle mass. No significant effect on weight, waist circumference, and BMI. (Morgentaler, et al., 2016)
- T treatment was associated with a significant increase in HGB (0.8 grams) and a decrease in HDL 0.49. There was no significant effect on mortality, prostate or CV outcomes.
- Androgen deprivation therapy-increase lipids and unfavorable lipid profile.
- Abnormal lipid profiles (higher total cholesterol, LDL, TG and lower HDL), elevation of pro-inflammatory factors, HTN, insulin resistance and endothelial dysfunction are common features in men with androgen deficiency.
- Causing or worsening of sleep apnea is frequently listed among potential adverse effects of testosterone replacement therapy, based primarily on case reports. Meta-analysis of 19 clinical trials through 2005 by Calof et al. showed no significant increase in obstructive sleep apnea; however, the studies were not conducted with polysomnography. The one study using this technique was performed by Hoyos et al., who treated middle-aged men who had severe obstructive sleep apnea with T. T mildly worsened sleep-disordered breathing after 7 weeks of treatment, but not after 18 weeks (Borst & Yarrow, 2015).
- T might protect against diabetes by a mechanism unrelated to cardiovascular disease. Testosterone builds muscle which provides a sink for glucose disposal and decreases fat mass.
- Acute administration of T at physiological concentrations directly into coronary vessels in men at cardiac catheterization increased coronary blood flow and coronary vasodilation in a dose-dependent manner. The

MORE SUPPORTIVE EVIDENCE FOR TESTOSTERONE

vasodilatory effects of T are mediated through L-type calcium channels explaining in part for the beneficial effect on angina.
- T deficiency is considered a pro-coagulant state. It exhibits decreased tissue plasminogen activator, increased fibrinogen, increased plasminogen activator inhibitor type 1 activity and increased thromboxane
- T use in the United States increased more than threefold between 2000 and 2011 (Borst & Yarrow, 2015)
- Age is accompanied by a decrease in both the number and diameter of muscle fibers, especially type II (fast) fibers. Fiber loss with aging is secondary to a loss in motor neurons. Testosterone replacement therapy increases muscle mass and strength by increasing the cross-sectional area of both type I and type II fibers in a dose-dependent manner (Borst & Yarrow, 2015).
- Fink et al. reported that the prevalence of osteoporosis in hypogonadal males was twice that of men with normal testosterone levels (6% vs 2.8%) (Cunningham & Toma, 2011)
- Basurto, et al. (2008) found that 12 months of T therapy increased spine and total hip BMD (bone mineral density) in men aged 60 years-old or older with serum T levels less than 320 ng/dl. (Kim S. , 2014)
- Long-acting Testosterone undecanoate in middle-aged men with late onset hypogonadism (T less than 320) significantly increased spine and femoral BMD after 3 years (Kim S. , 2014).
- A 2011 randomized controlled trial with 36 women with pre-existing cardiovascular disease in the form of severe congestive heart failure were randomly assigned to treatment

with transdermal testosterone or placebo for 6 months. Women given testosterone had significant improvements in the 6-minute walk test, oxygen consumption, and insulin resistance compared with those given placebo (Davis & Wahlin-Jacobsen, 2015).
- Hyper-androgenism in women because of polycystic ovary syndrome or high-dose angdrogen therapy in femalt-to-male trassexuals does not increase the risk of breast cancer (Dimitrakakis & Bondy, 2009).

Testosterone deficiency and cardiovascular mortality. Review of literature

Current evidence does not support the belief that T therapy is associated with increased CV risk or CV mortality. On the contrary, a wealth of evidence accumulated over several decades suggests that low T levels increase risk and normal to higher normal levels appear to be beneficial for CV mortality and risk (Morganteler, 2015).

Testosterone deficiency is associated with increased risk of mortality and testosterone replacement improves survival in men with type 2 diabetes

A total of 581 men with type 2 diabetes were followed for a mean period of 5.8 years. Mortality rates were compared between T levels above 300 ng/dl and below 300 ng/dl. Mortality was increased in the low T group (17.2%) compared with the normal T group (9%) when controlled for covariates. When data was reviewed in those who received T for 1 year or longer, a beneficial effect was found. The data showed that the survival curve followed a similar course to that of the normal T group, whereas the untreated group had a worse prognosis. **The increase in mortality was found to be independent of age, glycemic control, BMI, pre-existing CVD, current smoking status and treatment with either statins, ACEI or ARB at baseline** (Muraleedharan, Marsh, Kapoor, Channer, & Jones, 2013).

Low serum testosterone and increased mortality in men with coronary heart disease

Longitudinal follow-up study in tertiary referral cardiothoracic center. 930 consecutive men with coronary disease referred for diagnostic angiography recruited between June 2000 and June 2002 and followed for a mean of 6.9 +/- 2.1 years. The overall prevalence of T deficiency using bio-available T was 20.9%, using total T was 16.9% and using either was 24%. Excess mortality was noted in the androgen-deficient group compared to normal T Group (21% to 12%.)

The only parameters found to influence time to all-cause and vascular mortality were the presence of left ventricular dysfunction, aspirin therapy, B-blocker therapy and low serum bio-T (Malkin, et al., 2010). This is reassuring since it agrees with conventional important points towards evaluating and treating heart disease and potemtially adds a new risk factor to help stratify patients.

Testosterone Replacement Therapy and Mortality in Older men.

Key Points- There is a high level of evidence that hypogonadism is associated with increased all-cause mortality and reduced quality of life. There is a considerable body of credible evidence over several decades that testosterone replacement therapy (TRT) according to expert guidelines is safe and efficacious for men suffering from confirmed testosterone deficiency. There is emerging evidence that TRT in such cases of established hypogonadism may reduce all-cause mortality. Recent studies suggesting that TRT may increase cardiovascular risk are severely flawed and do not exclude the possibility that increased risk is related to hypogonadism and not the treatment (Hackett G. , 2016).

Elderly men over 65 years of age with late-onset hypogonadism benefit as much from testosterone treatment as do younger men.

Men over 65 benefit as much as younger men with testosterone replacement therapy and that benefit is lost when treatment is discontinued. **Maximum effects were observed after 12 months of treatment and up to 5 years** (Saad, Yassin, Haider, Doros, & Gooren, 2015).

Testosterone related good neurologic outcome on the patients with return of spontaneous circulation after cardiac arrest: a prospective cohort study.

Abstract
AIM:
To evaluate the gonadal hormones in patients with return of spontaneous circulation (ROSC) after cardiac arrest following prospectively good (cerebral-performance category [CPC] 1-2) and poor (CPC 3-5) neurologic outcomes.

METHODS:
The patients in an emergency center who had been admitted to the center's intensive care unit (ICU) after successful resuscitation following out-of-hospital cardiac arrest were prospectively identified and evaluated within the period from April 2008 to March 2011.

RESULTS:
A total of 142 patients were analyzed in this study. Thirty-nine (27.5%) patients had good neurologic outcomes. In the multiple logistic-regression analysis, the initial shockable rhythm, time from arrest to ROSC, and more than 300 ng/dl of testosterone level was found to be related to good neurologic outcome, respectively.

CONCLUSION:
Higher testosterone levels are related to good neurologic outcome at six months after admission in patients with spontaneous circulation after cardiac arrest. The testosterone levels may be useful prognostic tools for the postcardiac-arrest syndrome and could be used for the latter's neuroprotective treatment, but additional randomized controlled studies are needed (Kim, et al., 2013)

Testosterone deficiency increases hospital readmission and mortality rates in male patients with heart failure

110 hospitalized male patients with a left ventricular ejection fraction less than 45% and New York Heart Association classification IV had total testosterone and free testosterone levels drawn. Hypogonadism was defined as a total testosterone level less than 300 ng/dl and free testosterone level less than 10 ng/dl. 66 patients were

hypogonadal and 44 were not. Length of stay was longer in the low T group at 37 days compared to 25 days in the normal T group. The cumulative hazard of readmission within one year was 44% in the low T group compared to 22% in the normal T group. **Low testosterone level is an independent risk factor for hospital readmission within 90 days and increased mortality** (Santos, et al., 2015).

Clinical review: Endogenous testosterone and mortality in men: a systematic review and meta-analysis

21 studies were included in the review and 12 were eligible for meta-analysis which involved 16,184 subjects. Mean age was 61 years old with T level of 487 ng/dl. and mean follow-up time was 9.7 years.

Conclusion: Low endogenous testosterone levels are associated with increased risk of all-cause and CVD death in community based studies of men, but considerable between-study heterogeneity occurred. **A criticism is the mean T level was much higher than the typical 300 ng/dl used to define hypogonadism** (Araujo, et al., 2011). A person in my office with a level of 487 ng/dl does not have hypogonadism.

Low concentrations of serum testosterone predict acute myocardial infarction in men with type 2 diabetes mellitus

1,109 subjects with mean age 62 +/- 12 years had testosterone and SHBG levels measured with a mean follow-up of 14.1 years (+/- 5.3). The prevalence of type 2 diabetes

MORE SUPPORTIVE EVIDENCE FOR TESTOSTERONE

at baseline was 10% in men and 7.5% in women. **A significant inverse association between testosterone level and acute myocardial infarction was found in men with type 2 diabetes. The association remained statistically significant even when traditional risk factors including waist-to-hip ratio, systolic blood pressure, total cholesterol, and active smoking are factored in** (Daka, et al., 2015).

American Association of Clinical Endocrinologists and American College of Endocrinology Position Statement on the Association of Testosterone and Cardiovascular Risk

Recent reports related testosterone treatment to increased cardiovascular events. However, **there is no compelling evidence that testosterone therapy either increases or decreases cardiovascular risk**. Large-scale prospective randomized controlled trials on testosterone therapy, focusing on cardiovascular benefits and risks, are clearly needed. As with therapeutics in general, common sense, experience, and an individualized approach are recommended. I was working on a short paper for my areas quarterly medicine magazine on testosterone and the editor emailed me to hold-off submitting the article at that time due to these erroneous warnings. Accurate information is always paramount.

Data suggest that T levels in the mid-normal range relate to an optimal CV risk profile at any age, and that T levels either above or below the physiological normal range may increase the risk of atherosclerotic heart disease (Goodman, et al., 2015).

Type 2 diabetes mellitus and testosterone: a meta-analysis study

Demonstrated that T replacement therapy significantly improves HgbA1c in addition to fasting plasma glucose. It is reasonable to assume that T causes improvement in glycemic control at least in part by its positive effects on visceral adiposity (Corona, et al., 2010)(Corona, et al., 2010).

Testosterone Deficiency in Men: Systematic Review and Standard Operating Procedures for Diagnosis and Treatment

Testosterone preparations
1. Methyltestosterone, fluoxy-testosterone (oral pills)-the ingested hormone is almost completely inactivated by its first pass through the liver and has potential hepatotoxicity (hepatocellular adenoma, cholestasis, jaundice and hemorrhagic liver cysts). These formulations should no longer be used.
    The only safe oral formulation is Testosterone Undecanoate. Its absorption is variable and needs to be taken three times per day. Burn units have a tradition of using this formulation.
2. Transbuccal T avoids intestinal bypass/liver inactivation. Requires twice a day application under the tongue.
3. Transdermal preparation- gels or patches. Delivers 5 to 10 mg of T per day. My office experience has been variable absorption with decreasing effectiveness as BMI increases.

4. Subdermal pellets. Prolonged period of action but requires minor procedure to be placed under skin. Expensive.
5. Injectable (IM, SQ) can be given SQ twice per week, once per week or IM every week or 2 weeks. Testosterone cypionate or enanthate is 75-100 mg per week or 150-200 mg every 2 weeks respectively. Cypionate has a half- life of 8 days and enanthate has a half-life of 6-7 days. Cypionate is used more often in the USA. Injections may induce supra-physiological peak levels for 2-5 days followed by rapid decline to sub-physiological levels before next dose. The initial supra-physiological levels promote the rapid increase in hematocrit seen with this formulation. Patients may sometimes feel differently when levels are supra-physiological compared to levels right before the next shot. The younger the person, the more likely to notice the difference. The long-acting Testosterone Undecanoate shows a more favorable kinetic profile with levels in the mid normal range for about 12 weeks. This requires only 4-5 injections of 1000 mg per year. The average price in Fort Wayne, Indiana on June 2017 for 750 mg was just over $1000 at several pharmacies.

Testosterone can be converted to estradiol by aromatization or to DHT (dihydrotestosterone) by 5-alpha reductase. DHT is not suited for long-term therapy since DHT cannot be converted to estradiol which is necessary for bone health. DHEA is also not recommended for T therapy because it is felt ineffective in men.

A possible cause of obesity-induced T deficiency may be the increased estrogen that obesity promotes which exerts a negative feedback to the hypothalamic-pituitary axis and therefore decreasing LH release to the Leydig cells of the testes.

Although a history of prostate cancer has been considered an absolute contraindication to T therapy, this point is now under debate, at least for men deemed cured. 221 men who received either radical prostatectomy (179), brachytherapy (31), or radiotherapy (11) T therapy started 2.5 months to 8.5 years after definitive treatment and the duration of T therapy ranged from 3.3 months to 9 years. The total follow-up after starting T therapy exceeded 5,000 months (mean 22.67 months). No clinical recurrence was observed and only one patient had PSA recurrence (after 12 months of transdermal T and 17 months post-radical prostatectomy). Patients must be very symptomatic with hypogonadal complaints, tumor must be contained within the prostate and the Gleason score must not be high grade. Informed consent must be obtained and the patient must know that long term safety data is limited before consideration of T therapy. There are no compelling data to suggest that T therapy exacerbates lower urinary tract symptoms or promotes acute urinary retention. **If adequate T levels are obtained and the person does not have resolution or improvement in hypogonadal symptoms after 6 months of treatment, then treatment should be discontinued. Monitoring of several parameters are important. A baseline low T level should be obtained along with PSA, DRE (digital rectal exam), HGB or HCT before starting T therapy. A simple** very conservative approach is to check PSA, HGB/HCT, and T level at 3 months, 6 months, 12 months and then annually along with DRE at 6 months, 12 months and annually. PSA recommendations are mainly for men over 40 (Buvat J, 2013).

The Role of Androgens and Estrogens on Healthy Aging and Longevity

Approximately 20% of men older than 60 years and 50% of men older than 80 years have serum testosterone concentrations below the normal range for young men. Not only does the loss of testosterone negatively affect muscle mass in older men, it appears to also increase the risk of osteoporosis and fractures further contributing to increased morbidity and mortality in older men. Testosterone levels in women decline in the fourth decade of life and prior to menopause approach 50% of those seen in the third decade. **Upon completion of menopause, average concentrations of testosterone in women are approximately 15% of premenopausal levels**. Women have about four times the amount of estrogens compared with men. The meta-analysis of Greising and colleagues (2009) showed that postmenopausal women on estrogen hormone therapy had greater physical strength than those without treatment. Another study of twins showed that the sibling receiving estrogen therapy had greater muscle power and maximal walking speed than the treatment naïve twin (2009). During the first year of menopause, women lose an average 80% per year of their estrogens. **They exhibit an accelerated decline**

in muscle mass and strength around the time of the menopause. It is thought that estrogens influence indices of muscle damage and repair. Estrogens play a role in regulation of bone mass and strength by controlling activity of bone-forming osteoblasts and inhibiting activity and vitality of bone-resorbing osteoclasts. **Serum levels of both estrogens and androgens decrease with age and are inversely associated with the risk of fracture in aging men.** Physiological testosterone therapy has shown to improve vasodilatation and decrease diastolic blood pressure in women. Undesirable effects of prolonged postmenopausal exposure to estrogen replacement are increased risk of cancer and increased rates of venous thromboembolism and biliary tract surgery. (Horstman, Dillon, Urban, & Sheffield-Moore, 2012)

Why is Androgen Replacement in Males Controversial?

Treatment of testosterone deficiency due to diseases such as mumps, Kallmann syndrome, hypopituitarism, traumatic brain injury, etc. has been accepted and treated for decades without any large multicenter controlled studies documenting efficacy and safety. Many types of insulins have never been studied in controlled trials in pregnant women but it is used routinely in pregnancy. Levels of testosterone decrease by 1-2 % per year starting in our thirties. Levels decrease regardless of race also. Until recently, it was thought that testosterone deficiency in middle-aged men and older men mainly affected the quality of life, but it was unlikely to affect morbidity or mortality. However, population-based studies show that testosterone deficiency predicts future development of type 2 diabetes, metabolic syndrome, cardiovascular events, mobility limitations, frailty, sarcopenia and mortality. Libido decreases with levels less than 432 ng/dl, depression and diabetes type 2 are more common with testosterone levels below 288 ng/dl and erectile dysfunction is aggravated when levels are low below 230 ng/dl. Testosterone clearly does more for libido than erectile dysfunction. Erectile dysfunction is really a vascular disease rather than a low testosterone issue. Erectile medicines like Viagra, Cialis, Levitra affect blood flow and were initially developed for blood pressure control not erectile dysfunction. The European Male Ageing Study emphasized an important point by defining late-onset hypogonadism not only by using a testosterone level below 320 ng/dl as the cut-off level but requiring the presence of at least three sexual symptoms. It looked at a database of 3,359 men between 40 to 79 years of age. I think the best clinical definition of hypogonadism should not only include a certain T level but also symptoms that have a moderate to excellent correlation with low levels. Unfortunately, many symptoms are general and could be attributed to many issues.

A general recommendation is to image the pituitary for tumors if a total testosterone level is below 150 ng/dl. This sounds like a reasonable idea but it is based on one report that found six subjects with a macroadenoma or hypothalamic lesion out of a group of 164 men aged 27 to 79 years whose chief complaint was erectile dysfunction. Their T level was 104 ng/dl or less. When overweight or obese patients lose weight many times their testosterone level will increase indicating that their hypothalamic-pituitary-adrenal axis still works well. Fink et al. (1991) reported the prevalence of osteoporosis was twice as high in men with a low T level compared to normal level (6% vs 2.8%). No fracture data was done. Testosterone therapy promotes sebum production which increase acne and can accelerate male pattern baldness (androgenic alopecia is genetic predisposition to DHT antagonizing hair follicle). Testosterone treatment can aggravate sleep apnea by decreasing a person's response to hypercapnia but evidence is not very impressive and the real concern in my viewpoint is to avoid significant polycythemia. Sleep apnea that is not controlled will promote polycythemia from inadequate oxygen levels. Testosterone injections will have some initial supra-physiological levels thus stimulating erythropoiesis. If testosterone is started on a person with poorly controlled sleep apnea or untreated sleep apnea, monitoring Hgb level is important. Testosterone treatment will suppress gonadotropins and spermatogenesis and should not be given to testosterone-deficient men who desire to father a child in the future. This article reaffirmed the clear evidence that testosterone does not cause prostate cancer. What is interesting is serum testosterone levels decrease with age while prostate cancer increases substantially with age. Most doctors believe if you live long enough you will have clinical or subclinical prostate cancer (Cunningham & Toma, 2011). The answer regarding improving cognition and testosterone is unclear with mixed results. We know that exercise improves cognition and memory and if testosterone encourages someone to exercise, one could say that testosterone helps people indirectly in this regard.

Testosterone dose-response relationships in healthy young men.

Testosterone regulates many physiological processes and each process may have different dose-response relationships. To determine the effects of graded doses of T on body composition, muscle size, strength, power, sexual and cognitive functions, PSA, plasma lipids, hemoglobin, and insulin-like growth factor I (IGF-I) 61 eugonadal men, 18-35 years old were randomized to one of five groups to receive monthly injections of a long-acting gonadotropin-releasing hormone (GnRH) agonist, to suppress endogenous testosterone secretion, and weekly injections of 25, 50, 125, 300, 600 mg of testosterone enanthate for 20 weeks. By suppressing endogenous testosterone with GnRH, testosterone levels are controlled based on injection doses. Nadir T levels drawn before a new dose resulted in concentrations of 253 ng/dl for 25 mg, 306 for 50 mg, 542 for 125 mg, 1345 for 300 mg, and 2370 for 600 mg doses. Remember a level of 300 ng/dl requires T supplementation and 600 ng/dl is the desired therapeutic level.

Leg power was measured because power in the lower extremity is strongly related to performance of functional activities in the elderly. The changes in fat-free mass were highly dependent on T dose. Changes in leg press strength, leg power, thigh and quadriceps muscle volumes, hemoglobin, and IGF-I were positively correlated with T concentrations, whereas changes in fat mass and plasma HDL were negatively correlated. Sexual function, visual-spatial cognition, mood, and PSA did not change significantly at any dose. By prioritizing the goals of T therapy, we can better choose desired levels making it potentially safer to use. (Bhasin, et al., 2001)

The study showed essentially dose-response effect and showed that young men tolerated much higher doses than typical replacement doses for 20 weeks.

Effects of long-term treatment with testosterone on weight and waist size in 411 hypogonadal men with obesity classes I-III: observational data from two registry studies.

Abstract

BACKGROUND/OBJECTIVES:

Long-term testosterone replacement therapy (TRT) up to 5 years has been shown to produce progressive and sustainable weight loss (WL) in hypogonadal men. This study investigated effects of long-term TRT up to 8 years in hypogonadal men with different obesity classes.

SUBJECTS/METHODS:

Two independent observational registries we identified a total of 411 obese, hypogonadal men receiving TRT in urological clinics. The effects of TRT on anthropometric as well as metabolic parameters were studied for a maximum duration of 8 years, mean follow-up: 6 years. All men received long-acting injections of testosterone undecanoate in 3-monthly intervals.

RESULTS:

In all three classes of obesity, T therapy produced significant WL, decrease in waist circumference (WC) and body mass index (BMI).

In patients with class I obesity, mean weight decreased from 102.6 to 84.1 kg, change from baseline: -17.4 kg and -16.8%. WC in this group of patients decreased from 106.8 to 95.1 cm, change from baseline: -10.6 cm. BMI decreased from 32.69 to 27.07 change from baseline: -5.52 kg m (-2).

In patients with class II obesity, weight decreased from 116.8 to 91.3 kg, change from baseline: -25.3 kg and -21.5%. WC decreased from 113.5 to 100.0 cm, change from baseline: -13.9 cm. BMI decreased from 37.32 to 29.49, change from baseline: -8.15 kg m (-2).

In patients with class III obesity, weight decreased from 129.0 to 98.9 kg, change from baseline: -30.5 kg and -23.6%. WC decreased from 118.5 to 103.8 cm, change from baseline: -14.3 cm. BMI decreased from 41.93 to 32.46, change from baseline -9.96 kg m (-2).
CONCLUSIONS:
Testosterone therapy appears to be an effective approach to achieve sustained WL in obese hypogonadal men irrespective of severity of obesity. Based on these findings we suggest that T therapy offers safe and effective treatment strategy of obesity in hypogonadal men. (Saad F, 2016)

Injection of testosterone may be safer and more effective than transdermal administration for combating loss of muscle and bone in older men.

Administered T is partially converted to estradiol by the enzyme aromatase or to DHT (dihydrotestosterone) by 5 alpha-reductase. Injected T increases DHT by 2.2- fold and transdermal (patch or gel) elevates DHT 5.46-fold. DHT binds to androgen receptors with three times the affinity compared with T and DHT may mediate several of the adverse effects of T. Finasteride, a specific inhibitor of 5 alpha-reductase blocks conversion of T to DHT which may lessen any T adverse effects such as increasing prostate volume without interfering in increases in lean mass or muscle strength. **Finasteride added to T therapy may be a simple combination that improves compliance in older men.** Exercise and T therapy have additive benefits for muscle mass. T therapy may also increase the motivation to exercise in older men. For men unable to exercise, T therapy provides a means for increasing muscle mass without exercising. (Borst & Yarrow, 2015)

Insulin Resistance and Inflammation in Hypogonadotropic Hypogonadism and Their Reduction After Testosterone Replacement in Men with Type 2 Diabetes.

One-third of men with type 2 diabetes have hypogonadotrophic hypogonadism (HH). The study consisted of 94 men with type 2 diabetes (50 eugonadal, 44 men with HH). Men with HH were randomized to receive 250 mg Testosterone IM or placebo every 2 weeks for 24 weeks. Men with HH were noted to have higher subcutaneous and visceral fat mass than eugonadal men.

There was a decrease in subcutaneous fat mass (3.3 kg) and increase in lean mass (3.4 kg) after T administration. Visceral and hepatic fat did not change. Testosterone treatment also caused a significant fall in circulating concentrations of free fatty acids, C-reactive protein, interleukin-1B, tumor necrosis factor-alpha, and leptin.

Conclusion: Testosterone treatment in men with type 2 diabetes and HH increases insulin sensitivity, increases lean mass, and decreases subcutaneous fat (Dhindsa, et al., 2016).

Effects of testosterone on lean mass gain in elderly men: systematic review with meta-analysis of controlled and randomized studies.

Meta-analysis of randomized controlled studies looking at testosterone replacement therapy in men over 60 years of age with normal to low total testosterone levels (less than 550 ng/dl). A total of 651 elderly men with mean age of 65 to 77 years received testosterone from 12 weeks to 36 months or placebo (356 testosterone, 295 placebo). Lean mass increased from 1.65 to 6.20 kg. Fat mass decreased by approximately 1.78 kg.

Weakness of study is that 550 ng/dl is a normal testosterone level and this was more a supplementation dose than replacement dose (Neto, et al., 2015).

Osteoporotic Fractures in Men (MrOs) Study.

2,416 Swedish men aged 69-81 years old. 485 cardiovascular events including hospitalizations and deaths from coronary and cerebrovascular events occurred over a median 5 years of follow-up. Men with total testosterone in the highest quintile of values had a 30% lower risk of experiencing a cardiovascular event compared to men with testosterone in the lowest quintile. No association with estrogen was noted. (Ohlsson C, et al., 2011)

Low-dose transdermal testosterone therapy improves angina threshold in men with chronic stable angina: A randomized, double-blind, placebo-controlled study.

Experimental studies suggest that androgens induce coronary vasodilatation. 46 men with stable angina completed a 2-week, single-blind, placebo run-in, followed by double-blind randomization to 5 mg testosterone daily by transdermal patch or matching placebo for 12 weeks. Active treatment resulted in a 2-fold increase in androgen levels and a statistically significant increase in times on treadmill to 1-mm ST-segment depression from 309 seconds at baseline to 343 seconds at 4 weeks to 361 seconds after 12 weeks. (52 seconds difference vs 26 seconds in placebo group). The magnitude of the response was greater in those with lower baseline bioavailable T levels (English, Steeds, Jones, Diver, & Channer, 2000).

Men with testosterone deficiency and a history of cardiovascular diseases benefit from long-term testosterone therapy: observational, real-life data from a registry study

Long-term testosterone therapy (TTh) in men with hypogonadism has been shown to improve all components of the metabolic syndrome. We investigated the effects of long-term TTh up to 8 years in hypogonadal men with a history of cardiovascular disease (CVD).

In two urological clinics, we identified 77 hypogonadal men receiving TTh who also had a history of CVD. The effects of TTh on anthropometric and metabolic parameters were investigated up to 8 years. Any major adverse cardiovascular events were reported. All men received testosterone undecanoate at 3-monthly intervals.

We observed a significant weight loss and a decrease in waist circumference and body mass index.

Mean weight decreased from 114±13 kg to 91±9 kg, change from baseline: -24 kg and -20.2%.

Waist circumference decreased from 112 cm to 99 cm, change from baseline: -13 cm.

BMI decreased from 37 to 29, change from baseline: -8

Cardio-metabolic parameters such as lipid pattern, glycemic control, blood pressure, heart rate, and pulse pressure all improved significantly and sustainably. No patient suffered a major adverse cardiovascular event.
CONCLUSION:
In men with hypogonadism, long-term testosterone therapy appears to be effective in achieving sustained improvements in all cardiometabolic risk factors and may be effective as an add-on measure in the secondary prevention of cardiovascular events in hypogonadal men with a history of CVD (Haider, et al., 2016).

Testosterone replacement in hypogonadal men with angina improves ischemic threshold and quality of life

10 men average age 60.8 years received T for one month. Time to 1 mm ST depression increased by 53 seconds, mood scores improved, total cholesterol, and TNF alpha decreased.

Prospective studies clearly demonstrate that T treatment over 3 and 12 months improve symptoms as determined by NYHA class of heart failure, mood, functional exercise capacity and VO2 max (oxygen consumption) (Malkin, et al., Testosterone replacement in hypogonadal men with angina improves ischemic threshold and quality of life, 2004).

Suppression of endogenous testosterone production attenuates the response to strength training: a randomized, placebo-controlled, and blinded intervention study

26 healthy young men were divided into 2 groups, one group had endogenous testosterone suppressed with GnRH analogue (Zoladex) and the other received placebo. Both groups exercised similarly for 8 weeks.

The study demonstrated that suppression of endogenous testosterone production attenuates the increase in lean mass, increases storage of fat, and abolishes the increase in muscle strength during strength training in normal young men. **We conclude that endogenous testosterone is of paramount importance for the muscular adaptation to strength training** (Kvorning, Andersen, Brixen, & Madsen, 2006). The key question is whether this finding can be extended to frail elderly men and even women to help manage/treat sarcopenia and sarcopenic obesity.

Risk of Myocardial Infarction in Older Men Receiving Testosterone Therapy.

Testosterone therapy for older men has increased substantially over the past decade. Using Medicare beneficiaries, 6,355 patients treated with at least 1 injection of testosterone were matched with a cohort of 19,065 testosterone nonusers and followed for 8 years regarding MI diagnoses. Each patient had a composite MI prognostic score tabulated and divided into MI risk quartiles. For men in the highest quartile of the MI prognostic score, testosterone therapy was associated with a reduced risk of MI, whereas there was no difference in risk for the first, second, and third quartiles. Older men treated with testosterone did not appear to have an increased risk of MI. **A dose-response analysis demonstrated no increased risk of MI according to estimated cumulative dose of testosterone** (Baillargeon, et al., 2014).

A view of geriatrics through hormones. What is the relation between andropause and well-known geriatric syndromes?

Total testosterone decreases annually by 0.4-1.0 % resulting to levels beneath the reference range in 20% of healthy men over 60 years-old and 30-50% over 80 years-old. Free T and Bioavailable T decrease even faster, probably due to the age related SHBG increase (SHBG binds T). Male hypogonadism requires the presence of both clinical symptoms and low serum T levels. Calculated Free T is mostly used to help diagnosis when Total T values are between 230 ng/dl and 300 ng/dl. After 50 years of age, the lifetime risk for a fracture is 51% for women and 20% for men. Higher T is related to higher ghrelin which stimulates growth hormone release. Robust evidence still lacks on the role of T treatment in prevention of dementia in healthy elderly or patients with mild cognitive impairment. Data supports a rather neutral effect of T treatment on lipids. **Most studies** suggest a rather positive effect of T on CV risk factors and cardiovascular disease. Androgen related activity seems erythropoietin independent and implicates hepcidin. High levels of T rapidly suppress hepcidin. **Hemoglobin increases as hepcidin decreases**. (Hepcidin, a liver polypeptide, induces a reduction of iron intestinal absorption. Hepcidin increases iron sequestration in the macrophages and reduces erythropoiesis).

Because of irrational safety concerns about testosterone replacement therapy, only 5% of hypogonadal men receive appropriate treatment in the US. Most studies agree that serious adverse effects are rare if guidelines are followed and T levels remain within the physiological range. Testosterone treatment is contraindicated in

1. Active prostate cancer.
2. Increasing PSA without urological assessment.
3. Severe lower urinary tract symptoms (International Prostate Symptom Score >19)
4. Hct >50% (relative). I would say 55-56%
5. Uncontrolled CHF or ischemic heart disease in the preceding 6 months.
6. Untreated severe obstructive sleep apnea.

(Samaras, et al., 2013)

Cardiovascular risk associated with testosterone-boosting medications: a systematic review and meta-analysis.

An up-to-date meta-analysis of random-controlled trials involving 75 studies with 3,016 men treated with testosterone and 2,448 with placebo for a mean duration of 34 weeks. **Testosterone supplementation was not associated with cardiovascular adverse events** (Corona, et al., 2014).

Injectable testosterone undecanoate for the treatment of hypogonadism.

Abstract
INTRODUCTION:
Injectable testosterone undecanoate (TU) is a long-acting testosterone (T) formulation available for the treatment of male hypogonadism (HG) since 2003.
AREAS COVERED:
The efficacy and safety of injectable TU are assessed, as obtained by meta-analyzing available evidence. An extensive Medline, Embase and Cochrane search was performed. All uncontrolled and placebo-controlled randomized clinical trials (RCTs), evaluating the effect of injectable TU on different outcomes, were included. Of the 98 retrieved articles, 33 were included in the study. Among those, 11 were placebo-controlled RCTs. Injectable TU was significantly associated with a reduction of fat mass and HbA1c in both controlled and uncontrolled trials, in particular when hypogonadal subjects were enrolled. Similar results were observed for the improvement of erectile function. In addition, TU ameliorated several other outcomes, including blood pressure, lipid profile, waist circumference and body mass index in uncontrolled studies, but these data were not confirmed in placebo-controlled trials. The treatment was well tolerated and no risk of prostate cancer or cardiovascular disease was observed.

EXPERT OPINION:

Injectable TU is a safe and effective treatment for male HG. The possibility of a therapeutic intervention just four to five times per year frees the patient, at least partially, from having a chronic condition, thus maintaining a positive, active role in self-caring. (Corona, Maseroli, & Maggi, 2014)

Effect and safety of testosterone undecanoate in the treatment of late-onset hypogonadism: a meta-analysis.

Abstract

OBJECTIVE:

To evaluate the efficacy and safety of testosterone undecanoate (TU) in the treatment of late-onset hypogonadism (LOH) by meta-analysis.

RESULTS:

14 studies were included after screening, which involved 1,686 cases. Compared with the placebo and control groups, TU treatment significantly increased the levels of serum total testosterone and serum free testosterone but decreased the contents of luteinizing hormone, sex hormone binding globulin. TU also remarkably reduced the scores of Partial Androgen Deficiency of the Aging Males and Aging Males Symptoms rating scale but increased the hemoglobin level. However, no significant changes were shown in aspartate aminotransferase, alanine transaminase, prostate-specific antigen, or prostate volume after TU treatment ($P > 0.05$).

CONCLUSION:
TU could significantly increase the serum testosterone level and improve the clinical symptoms of LOH patients without inducing serious adverse reactions. However, due to the limited number and relatively low quality of the included studies, the above conclusion could be cautiously applied to clinical practice. (Zheng, et al., 2015)

The efficacy and safety of oxandrolone treatment for patients with severe burns: A systematic review and meta-analysis.

Abstract
OBJECTIVE:
The objective of this systematic review and meta-analysis was to evaluate the efficacy and safety of using oxandrolone in patients with severe burns.
RESULTS:
15 randomized controlled trials (RCTs) were identified for analysis in this review, including 806 participants.

Oxandrolone therapy did not affect mortality or infection. The two groups (oxandrolone group vs. control group) showed no significant difference in liver dysfunction.

All the 15 RCTs reported no incidence of hepatic insufficiency in controls or treatment groups.

In the catabolic phase: Treatment with oxandrolone significantly shortened length of stay by 3.02 days, donor-site healing time by 4.41 days, the time between surgical procedures by 0.63 days, as well as reduced weight loss by 5 kg and nitrogen loss by 8.19 g/day,

In the rehabilitative phase: Treatment with oxandrolone significantly shortened the length of stay to 6.45 days, as well as decreased weight loss by 0.86 kg/week and reduction of lean body mass by 5%.

Long-term parameters: Oxandrolone treatment led to a statistically significant additional gain in lean body mass of 3.99% after 6 months and 10.78% after 12 months in patients with severe burns, with all P<0.00001.
CONCLUSION:
The treatment of severe burns with oxandrolone is significantly effective without obvious side effects (Li, Guo, Yang, Roy, & Guo, 2016).

A criticism involves using an oral androgenic/anabolic steroid instead of IM or SQ testosterone. Oral steroids have to be given several times per day and can promote significant liver disease. I suspect oxandrolone was used due to tradition and past successful experience with it. I would think that an IM or SQ testosterone shot would still work well even in a burn patient.

A critical analysis of testosterone supplementation therapy and cardiovascular risk in elderly men.

Testosterone supplementation therapy should be used judiciously in elderly males, with a paradigm focused on returning serum T levels to normal limits, rather than treating with supra-physiological doses (Scovell, Ramasamy, & Kovac, 2014).

In older men, higher plasma testosterone or dihydrotestosterone are independent predictors for reduced incidence of stroke but not myocardial infarction.

3,690 men aged 70-89 years old followed for 6.6 years during which time 344 men experienced a MI and 300 men a stroke.

Higher baseline total testosterone or dihydrotestosterone was associated with lower incidence of stroke, but not MI. Estradiol was not associated with either outcome. The same 3,690 men were followed for 7.1 years during which time there were 974 deaths, 325 from ischemic heart disease.

Testosterone in the middle of the range was associated with lower overall mortality. Higher dihydrotestosterone was associated with lower Ischemic heart disease mortality (Yeap, et al., 2014).

Older Men Are as Responsive as Young Men to the Anabolic Effects of Graded Doses of Testosterone on the Skeletal Muscle.

Randomized, double-blind trial with 60 ambulatory, healthy, older men, 60-75 years of age with normal testosterone levels were compared with younger men 19-35 years old to graded doses of testosterone. Participants received a long-acting GNRH agonist to suppress endogenous testosterone to allow accurate reflections of the given testosterone doses. The men received weekly doses of 25, 50, 125, 300, and 600 mg testosterone enanthate for 20 weeks. **Hemoglobin levels were dose dependent**

and increased significantly greater in older men than young men. Changes in FFM (fat free mass) and muscle strength correlated with testosterone dose and were not significantly different in young and older men. **Older men are as responsive as young men to testosterone's anabolic effects.** Frequency of hematocrit greater than 54%, leg edema, and prostate events were numerically higher in older men than in younger men.

The best trade-off was achieved with a testosterone dose of 125 mg per week. The 125mg dose was associated with high-normal testosterone concentrations and low frequency of adverse events, no serious adverse events and substantial gains in FFM (+4.2 kg) and leg press strength (+28 kg). Gains in leg press strength in older men receiving 125, 300, and 600 mg doses averaged 28-50 kg gains. Thus, skeletal muscle in older men is capable of undergoing considerable hypertrophy in response to androgenic stimulus. Because supra-physiological doses of testosterone (300 and 600 mg) were associated with a high frequency of adverse events, it is unlikely that these doses can be used in long-term human trials. Leg edema developed in some older patients receiving 300 or 600 mg doses. **Sexual function did not change significantly at any dose in either age group. Testosterone dose-response relationships differ for different androgen-dependent outcomes: sexual function and PSA levels are maintained at lower testosterone concentrations than those required to induce muscle growth. We do not know whether testosterone-induced gains in muscle mass and strength translate into improved physical**

function, quality of life, or decreased fracture risk (Bhasin, et al., 2005).

Clinical Review: Testosterone Use in Men and Its Effects on Bone Health. A Systematic Review and Meta-analysis of Randomized Placebo-Controlled Trials.

Eight trials enrolling 365 patients. Two trials followed patients for more than 1 year. Testosterone was associated with an 8% gain in lumbar bone mineral density and transdermal testosterone had no significant impact. Testosterone use was associated with a nonsignificant 4% gain in femoral neck bone mineral density with unexplained differences in results across trials. No trials measured or reported the effect of testosterone on fractures. **Without bone fracture data, the available trials offer weak and indirect inferences about the clinical efficacy of testosterone on osteoporosis prevention and treatment in men**. Although testosterone seems to play an important role in bone maintenance and bone formation, it appears more likely that a complex interaction between testosterone and estrogen (through their respective receptors) is key in the regulation of the male bone skeleton such that testosterone may impact bone health indirectly and, perhaps to a greater extent, through aromatization to estrogen (Tracz, et al., 2006). From reading literature, it seems estrogen is key player for bone health.

Testosterone and Surgical Outcomes

WE CAN IMPROVE ANEMIA WITH testosterone along with decrease the strong catabolic stress that illness causes. Hopefully, testosterone can decrease transfusion rate, length of stay in the hospital or skilled nursing facility and improve some outcomes. Bedrest and the stress of surgery or illness can dramatically weaken a person and promote rapid muscle mass loss and strength. Some will recover from this insult and others will never recover from a serious medical insult. Testosterone may help but it is important to use responsible doses and the benefits are probably measured more in months and years than weeks. For testosterone to provide the best results, foresight is required giving the idea of early treatment protocols a necessary endeavor. For instance, a person having hip arthroplasty or multilevel fusion would need to start testosterone 4-6 weeks before surgery.

Prevalence of Total Hip and Knee Replacement in the United States.

The prevalence of total hip and total knee replacement in the U.S population in 2010;
Total hip 1.4 million women, 1.1 million men.
Total knee 3 million women, 1.7 million men.

A substantial rise in prevalence over time and a shift to younger ages.

In 2010, a little over 2% of the U.S. population were living with a total hip or total knee replacement. This corresponds to an estimated 7 million people. Total joint replacement is surprisingly more prevalent than several chronic diseases that catch the public's attention. Overall prevalence is similar to stroke (6.8 million) and myocardial infarction (7.6 million) and much higher than heart failure (5.1 million). Clearly, living with a total joint replacement is a remarkably common condition. (Maradit Kremers, et al., 2015). **Improving muscle mass with exercise and/or testosterone slows down the wear and tear of the joint by improving the strength of supportive structures.**

Systematic review and meta-analysis of the association between frailty and outcome in surgical patients

Frailty is becoming increasingly prevalent in the elderly population with no consensus definition present. An estimated prevalence in excess of 10% in community dwelling adults aged 65 years and over, and higher levels seen with increasing age and in women. A literature search with collated data from 12 studies revealed the following;

1. Higher in-hospital mortality rate-odds ratio 2.77 (i.e. 277% greater risk)
2. Higher one-year mortality rate-odds ratio 1.99
3. Longer hospital stay-odds ratio 1.05
4. Higher discharge rate to rehab/SNF-odds ratio 5.71

Cumulative co-morbidity may lead to poor outcome as patients may develop complications directly related to their medical condition or they may simply have reduced physiological reserve. (Oakland, Nadler, Cresswell, Jackson, & Coughlin, 2016).

It is unclear whether Testosterone therapy or IV iron therapy can help this type of patient but the upside seems worth any potential downside in my opinion.

Preoperative Supra-Physiological Testosterone in Older Men Undergoing Knee Replacement Surgery.

More than 100,000 knee replacements are performed yearly in the United States and 90% of these patients are aged 55 years or older.

Double-blind, placebo-controlled VA study involving 25 men, mean age 70 years, undergoing elective knee replacement received 600 mg Testosterone enanthate IM weekly 21, 14, 7, and 1 day before surgery. Testosterone levels were similar between treated and placebo patients before randomization.

1. Length of stay was not significantly lower in T group compared to placebo (5.9 days vs 6.7 days).
2. 20% required inpatient rehab in T group compared to 25% in placebo.
3. Three days after surgery, subjects in the T group stood significantly better than those who received placebo.
4. T group demonstrated a trend toward better FIM scores in walking and stair climbing (FIM is 7- point scale in which higher scores indicate greater function and independence).

5. By postoperative day 35, the overall FIM score had returned to baseline or better in 31% of T patients, compared with 18% of placebo.
6. There was a trend toward increased postoperative hematocrit in the T group on postoperative days 3 and 35 compared with placebo.
7. There were no significant changes in serum markers of kidney, liver, or PSA levels in either group.
8. An additional benefit of preoperative T might be a decreased need for blood transfusions because of the preoperative increase in hematocrit mediated by testosterone.

In summary, preoperative supra-physiological T administration to older men undergoing knee replacement surgery appears to be safe and leads to improvements in some measures of postoperative recovery. The doses were 4-5 times the typical replacement dose with elderly men tolerating them (Amory, et al., 2002).

Association of Testosterone Levels with Anemia in Older Men: A Controlled Clinical Trial.

In one-third of older men with anemia, no recognized cause can be found.
OBJECTIVE:
To determine if testosterone treatment of men 65 years or older with unequivocally low testosterone levels and unexplained anemia would increase their hemoglobin concentration.

A double-blinded, placebo-controlled trial with 788 men 65 years or older who have average testosterone levels of less than 275 ng/dl. Of 788 participants, 126 were anemic (hemoglobin ≤12.7 g/dl), 62 of whom had no known cause. The trial was conducted in 12 academic medical centers in the United States from June 2010 to June 2014.

INTERVENTIONS:

Testosterone gel, the dose adjusted to maintain the testosterone levels normal for young men, or placebo gel for 12 months.

MAIN OUTCOMES AND MEASURES:

The percent of men with unexplained anemia whose hemoglobin levels increased by 1.0 g/dl or more in response to testosterone compared with placebo.

RESULTS:

The men had a mean age of 74.8 years and BMI of 30.7; 84.9% were white. Testosterone treatment resulted in a greater percentage of men with unexplained anemia whose 12 month hemoglobin levels had increased by 1.0 g/dl or more over baseline (54%) than did placebo (15%) and a greater percentage of men who at month 12 were no longer anemic (58.3%) compared with placebo (22.2%) Testosterone treatment also resulted in a greater percentage of men with anemia of known cause whose month 12 hemoglobin levels had increased by 1.0 g/dl or more (52%) than did placebo (19%). Testosterone treatment resulted in a hemoglobin concentration of more than 17.5 g/dl in 6 men who had not been anemic at baseline.

CONCLUSIONS AND RELEVANCE:

Among older men with low testosterone levels, testosterone treatment significantly increased the hemoglobin levels of those with unexplained anemia as well as those with anemia from known causes. These increases may be of clinical value, as suggested by the magnitude of the changes and the correction of anemia in most men, but the overall health benefits remain to be established. Measurement of testosterone levels might be considered in men 65 years or older who have unexplained anemia and symptoms of low testosterone levels (Roy, et al., 2017).

Instead of just ordering a ferritin, iron profile and B12 level for anemia, we may want to add a total morning testosterone level also.

The relationship between serum total testosterone and free testosterone levels with serum hemoglobin and hematocrit levels: a study in 1221 men.

Investigate the relationship between serum total testosterone (TT) and free testosterone (FT) levels in men with anemia.

We reviewed the records of 1221 subjects between March 2009 and December 2014.
RESULTS:
The mean age was 59.8 years old. The mean TT and FT levels were 4.54 ng/ml and 10.63 ng/ml, respectively. The mean hemoglobin (Hgb) and hematocrit (Hct) levels were 14.72 g/dl and 43.11%, respectively. Subjects with low TT (<2.35 ng/mL) had low Hgb and Hct levels ($p<0.001$, $p<0.001$, respectively). TT was positively associated with FT, Hgb, and Hct. TT and FT levels were significantly lower in older men.

Subjects with low TT and FT levels had low Hgb and Hct levels. This suggests that TT and FT play a significant role in erythropoiesis. Testosterone replacement therapy may be effective in men with hypogonadism to reduce the incidence of anemia (Shin, You, Cha, & Park, 2016).

Could Testosterone Replacement Therapy in Hypogonadal Men Ameliorate Anemia, a Cardiovascular Risk Factor? An Observational, 54-Week Cumulative Registry Study.

Investigated if testosterone undecanoate attenuates anemia and the risk of cardiovascular disease in patients with hypogonadism.

MATERIALS AND METHODS:

A registry study consisted of 58 participants with a subnormal total testosterone level (less than 2.35 ng/ml) and at least mild symptoms of testosterone deficiency. All patients received an injection of 1,000 mg testosterone undecanoate at the initial visit, followed by injection at 6, 18, 30, 42 and 54 weeks. Serum hormones, hemoglobin, hematocrit, anemia risk factors, lipid profiles, whole blood viscosity and anthropometry were measured.

RESULTS:

Total testosterone (from mean 1.87 to 5.52 ng/ml, $p < 0.001$) and free testosterone (from 3.04 to 7.23 pg/ml, $p < 0.001$) were restored by testosterone undecanoate therapy. Hemoglobin and hematocrit significantly increased after testosterone undecanoate therapy by an average of 2.46 gm/dl ($p < 0.001$) and 3.03% ($p < 0.001$), respectively. The prevalence of anemia (from 29.6% to

10.0%) significantly decreased (p <0.001) and patients with anemia showed a significant increase in erythropoietin after testosterone undecanoate therapy (p = 0.047). A reduction in total cholesterol (from 165.89 to 153.80 mg/dl, p = 0.002), increased whole blood viscosity and increased hematocrit were observed until 54 weeks compared with baseline. However, whole blood viscosity and hematocrit stabilized after 18 weeks.

CONCLUSIONS:

After 54 weeks, testosterone undecanoate decreased the prevalence of anemia and components of the metabolic syndrome. A longer duration of testosterone undecanoate therapy of more than 18 weeks may be effective and safe in reducing blood viscosity and improving anemia (Zhang, Shin, Kim, & Park, 2016).

The cost of testosterone undecanoate is approximately $1000 for 750 mg at several pharmacies in Fort Wayne, Indiana on 6/9/2017. This is without any coupons or insurance discounts.

Transfusions and blood loss in total hip and knee arthroplasty: a prospective observational study.

There is a high prevalence of blood product transfusions in orthopedic surgery. The reported prevalence of red cell transfusions in unselected patients undergoing hip or knee replacement varies between 21% and 70%.

193 consecutive patients undergoing unilateral hip (114) or knee arthroplasty (79) were included in a prospective observational study.

Overall transfusion rate was 16% (18% in hip patients and 11% in knee patients). Preoperative hemoglobin concentration was the only independent predictor of red cell transfusion in hip patients, while low hemoglobin concentration, body mass index, and operation time were independent predictors for red cell transfusion in knee patients.

Low BMI was associated with an increased risk of excessive blood loss. This is in accordance with findings from heart surgery, where low BMI has been shown to be a risk for reoperation because of excessive bleeding. For hip arthroplasty, Bowditch & Villar (1999) reported an increased risk of bleeding in obese patients. (Carling, Jeppsson, Eriksson, & Brisby, 2015). **Using the erythrocytosis side effect of testosterone can be used to our advantage to lessen the need for transfusions for any surgery**

Effect of testosterone on hepcidin, ferroportin, ferritin, and iron binding capacity in patients with hypogonadotropic hypogonadism and type 2 diabetes.

The increase in hematocrit following testosterone therapy is associated with an increase in erythropoietin, the suppression of hepcidin, and an increase in the expression of ferroportin and transferrin receptor. Ferroportin and transferrin receptor are proteins that help transport iron and hepcidin decreases iron absorption (Dhindsa, et al., Effect of testosterone on hepcidin, ferroportin, ferritin, and iron binding capacity in patients with hypogonadotropic hypogonadism and type 2 diabetes, 2016).

Locomotive Syndrome: Definition and Management.

Locomotive syndrome is a condition of reduced mobility due to impairment of locomotive organs. The Japanese Orthopedic Association proposed the term in 2007. The average Japanese life expectancy in the year 2014 was 80.5 years for men and 86.8 years for women. Common issues among people aged 70-74 years old include fear of falling (81.7%), not being able to stand without arm support (81.1%), not being able to ascend stairs without using rail or wall for support (81.3%), slow gait speed (71.7%), and refraining from going out (50%). The three main components of the locomotive syndrome are

1. Bones, joints, intervertebral disks
2. Muscular system
3. Nervous system.

The orthopedic conditions contributing to the locomotive syndrome have high prevalence rates in patients above 40 years.

1. Lumbar spondylosis 81.5% males, 65.6% females
2. Knee osteoarthritis 42.6% males, 62.4% females
3. Osteoporosis 12.4% males, 26.5% females.
4. Sarcopenia 13.8% males, 12.4% females.

It is surprising to me how early pathology starts. The number of orthopedic surgical treatments requiring hospitalization dramatically increases after the age of 50 years. While physical interventions are effective in people with mild to moderate disability, their utility is limited in people with severe disability, emphasizing the importance of early detection of the locomotive syndrome and early intervention. (Nakamura & Ogata, 2016).

Testosterone treatment could be helpful in this situation by promoting supportive muscle mass, and increasing the number of years that a healthier orthopedic reserve could allow us to engage in leisure and fun activities

Androgen Therapy and Re-hospitalization in Older Men with Testosterone Deficiency.

A retrospective cohort of 6,372 nonsurgical hospitalizations looking at 30-day re-hospitalization rates comparing androgen users versus non-androgen users in men aged 66 years and older with a previous diagnosis of testosterone deficiency. The re-hospitalization rate was 9.8% (91 0f 929 androgen users) versus 13.0% (708 of 5,443 non-androgen users). Androgen therapy may reduce the risk of re-hospitalization in older men with testosterone deficiency and this intervention potentially holds broad clinical and public health relevance (Baillargeon, et al., 2016).

Testosterone Replacement Therapy and Bone Mineral Density in Men with Hypogonadism.

Men with hip fractures have a mortality rate two to three times higher than women. The risk of mortality one year post-fracture has been shown to be approximately 1.4 to 2.1 times higher in men than in women. Reports find that osteoporosis is underdiagnosed and undertreated in men. A secondary cause of osteoporosis is common in men, such as glucocorticoid excess, hypogonadism, or alcohol excess. Alcohol abuse is a worldwide issue with men associated with significant morbidity and mortality. People usually don't think of osteoporosis with alcoholism. Having weak bones and a higher incidence of falling from alcohol abuse can be a deadly nightcap.

Several studies (1999, 2006, 2007) found that men whose serum T level is 200-300 ng/dl or below are at higher risk for bone loss and fracture and have a favorable response to T treatment.

Men greater than 65 years-old with low T levels are at an increased risk of falls, osteoporosis and fractures. A controlled trial evaluated the effect of 36 months of T on bone health in men with late-onset hypogonadism: this study found substantial increases in both lumbar and femoral bone mineral density (Kim S. , 2014). The key question always with treating osteoporosis is fracture data.

Testosterone and Prostate

THE IDEA THAT TESTOSTERONE CAUSES prostate cancer has been conclusively shown to be not true. A 15-yr retrospective study of 150,000 men by Kaplan and Hu found that testosterone replacement therapy was not associated with prostate cancer. Meta-analysis by Calof et al. reported no evidence that T administration increases prostate cancer. Case closed. More and more literature is showing that testosterone replacement therapy is safe to use in surgically cured prostate cancer patients. Erectile dysfunction is probably the major reason that testosterone levels are checked. Erectile dysfunction is much more a vascular disease than a hormonal disease. Drugs such as Viagra, Cialis, Levitra work by vasodilation. Erectile medicines were discovered accidently as a side effect of medicines being studied to lower blood pressure. Testosterone gets one in the mood but the state of your vasculature system does the hard work. The following articles start in June 1996 discussing sildenafil as a promising drug till March 2017 showing its effectiveness despite age and comorbidities. Sildenafil has come a long way since its approval in March 27, 1998. (Borst & Yarrow, 2015)

Sildenafil: an orally active type 5 cyclic GMP-specific phosphodiesterase inhibitor for the treatment of penile erectile dysfunction.

Abstract

Sildenafil (Viagra, UK-92,480) is a novel oral agent under development for the treatment of penile erectile dysfunction. Erection is dependent on nitric oxide and its second messenger, cyclic guanosine monophosphate (cGMP). However, the relative importance of phosphodiesterase (PDE) isozymes is not clear. We have identified both cGMP- and cyclic adenosine monophosphate-specific phosphodiesterases (PDEs) in human corpora cavernosa in vitro. The main PDE activity in this tissue was due to PDE5, with PDE2 and 3 also identified. **Sildenafil is a selective inhibitor of PDE5**. In human volunteers, we have shown sildenafil to have suitable pharmacokinetic and pharmacodynamic properties (rapid absorption, relatively short half-life, no significant effect on heart rate and blood pressure) for an oral agent to be taken, as required, prior to sexual activity. Moreover, in a clinical study of 12 patients with erectile dysfunction without an established organic cause, we have shown sildenafil to enhance the erectile response (duration and rigidity of erection) to visual sexual stimulation, thus highlighting the important role of PDE5 in human penile erection. Sildenafil holds promise as a new effective oral treatment for penile erectile dysfunction. (Boolell, et al., 1996)

Sildenafil, a novel effective oral therapy for male erectile dysfunction.

Abstract

OBJECTIVES:

To determine the efficacy and safety of sildenafil, a novel orally active inhibitor of the type-V cyclic guanosine monophosphate-specific phosphodiesterase (the predominant isoenzyme in the human corpus cavernosum) on penile erectile activity in patients with male erectile dysfunction of no established organic cause.

PATIENTS AND METHODS:

Twelve patients (aged 36-63 years) with male erectile dysfunction of no established organic cause were entered into a double-blind, randomized, placebo-controlled, crossover study which was conducted in two phases. In the first phase (four-way crossover), treatment efficacy was evaluated by measurements of penile rigidity using penile plethysmography during visual sexual stimulation at different doses of sildenafil (10, 25 and 50 mg or placebo). In the second phase (two-way crossover), efficacy was assessed by a diary record of penile erectile activity after single daily doses of sildenafil (25 mg) or placebo for 7 days.

RESULTS:

The mean (95% confidence interval, CI) duration of rigidity of > 80% at the base of the penis was 1.3 min in patients on placebo, 3.5 min on 10 mg, 8.0 min on 25 mg and 11.2 min on 50 mg of sildenafil. The mean (95% CI) duration of rigidity of > 80% at the tip of the penis was 1.2 min on placebo and 7.4 min on 50 mg sildenafil. From the diary

record of daily erectile activity, the mean (95% CI) total number of erections was significantly higher in patients receiving sildenafil was 6.1 (3.2-11.4), compared with 1.3 (0.5-2.7) in those on placebo; 10 of 12 patients reported improved erectile activity while receiving sildenafil, compared with two of 12 on placebo (P = 0.018). Six patients on active treatment and five on placebo reported mild and transient adverse events which included headache, dyspepsia and pelvic musculo-skeletal pain.
CONCLUSION:
These results show that sildenafil is a well-tolerated and effective oral therapy for male erectile dysfunction with no established organic cause and may represent a new class of peripherally acting drug for the treatment of this condition. (Boolell, Gepi-Attee, Gingell, & Allen, 1996)

Treatment response to sildenafil in men with erectile dysfunction relative to concomitant comorbidities and age.

Abstract
AIM:
To evaluate treatment response in men with erectile dysfunction (ED) and concomitant comorbidities.
METHODS:
Data were pooled from 42 placebo-controlled, flexible-dose sildenafil trials. In most trials, the sildenafil dose was 50 mg, taken ~1 hour before sexual activity but not more than once daily, with adjustment to 100 or 25 mg as needed. The overall population (N=9413) was stratified by age (<45, 46-64, ≥65 years). Treatment response was defined as a minimal clinically important difference

(MCID) from baseline in the International Index of Erectile Function-Erectile Function (IIEF-EF) domain score of >2, >5 and >7 for men with mild, moderate and severe ED at baseline, respectively, or an IIEF-EF domain score ≥26 (no ED) at end-point.

RESULTS:

In the overall population, treatment response using the IIEF-EF MCID definition was significantly greater (P<.0001) with sildenafil vs placebo in men with no comorbidity (77% vs 33%), cardiovascular disease/hypertension only (71% vs 27%), diabetes only (63% vs 24%) or depression only (78% vs 29%). Using an IIEF-EF score ≥26, treatment response was significantly greater (P<.0001) with sildenafil vs placebo in men with no comorbidity (49% vs 17%), cardiovascular disease/hypertension only (48% vs 12%), diabetes only (40% vs 12%) or depression only (60% vs 17%). With each definition, the treatment response for each age and comorbidity was significantly greater (P≤.0065) with sildenafil vs placebo.

CONCLUSION:

The treatment response was significantly greater with sildenafil vs placebo in men with ED and each comorbidity regardless of age. (Goldstein, Stecher, & Carlsson, 2017)

Combined testosterone and vardenafil treatment for restoring erectile function in hypogonadal patients who failed to respond to testosterone therapy alone.

Abstract

INTRODUCTION:

The role of testosterone in erectile dysfunction (ED) is increasingly recognized. It is suggested that assessment of testosterone deficiency in men with ED and symptoms of hypogonadism, prior to first-line treatment, may be a useful tool for improving therapy.

AIM:

In this prospective, observational, and longitudinal study, we investigated the effects of vardenafil (Levitra) treatment as adjunctive therapy to testosterone undecanoate in hypogonadal ED patients who failed to respond to testosterone treatment alone.

METHODS:

One hundred twenty-nine testosterone deficient (serum total testosterone ≤ 340 ng/dL) patients aged 56 ± 3.9 years received intramuscular injections of long-acting parenteral testosterone undecanoate at 3-month intervals for 8 months mean follow-up.

MAIN OUTCOME MEASURES:

Scores on the International Index of Erectile Function Questionnaire-five items (IIEF-5) and partner survey scores were compared at baseline and posttreatment with testosterone therapy alone or in combination with vardenafil. Patient baseline demographics and concomitant disease were correlated with patients' IIEF-5 scores.

RESULTS:

Seventy-one (58.2%) responded well to monotherapy within 3 months. Nonresponders had lower testosterone levels and higher rates of concomitant diseases and smoking. Thirty-four of the 51 nonresponders accepted the addition of 20 mg vardenafil on demand. Efficacy assessments were measured by the IIEF-erectile function domain (IIEF-EF, questions 1-5 plus 15, 30 points) and partner self-designed survey at baseline after 4-6 weeks and at study end point. Thirty out of 34 patients responded well to this combination. IIEF-EF Sexual Health Inventory for Men score improved from 12 to 24 (P < 0.0001), and partner survey showed significantly higher satisfaction (P < 0.001). These patients reported spontaneous or nocturnal and morning erections or tumescence. No changes in adverse effects were recorded.

CONCLUSIONS:

These data suggest that combination therapy of testosterone and vardenafil is safe and effective in treating hypogonadal ED patients who failed to respond to testosterone monotherapy. (Yassin DJ, 2014)

Patient satisfaction with testosterone replacement therapies: the reasons behind the choices.

Anonymous, prospective survey given to men taking T at an academic urology clinic. Average age 49 years-old (382 patients); 53% received injections, 31% gels, 17% pellets. Satisfaction rates between 6-12 months were 68% gel, 73%injections, 70% pellets. **Satisfied patients reported improvements in the domains of energy, libido, concentration, mood, and muscle mass at a significantly higher rate than patients who were dissatisfied** (Kovac, et al., 2014).

Testosterone replacement therapy and voiding dysfunction.

The current evidence suggests that not only does testosterone replacement therapy not worsen lower urinary tract symptoms (LUTS), but that hypogonadism itself is an important risk factor for lower urinary tract symptoms and benign prostatic hyperplasia (Baas & Köhler, 2016).

Testosterone deficiency and severity of erectile dysfunction are independently associated with reduced quality of life in men with type 2 diabetes.

Erectile dysfunction and low T levels are common in men with type 2 diabetes. Men with ED were identified within a study cohort of 355 men with TD2. Men completed the SF-36 (short-form 36 question health survey with good reliability), and had total T, bio-T, and calculated free T drawn. The SF-36 scores significantly and positively correlated with all three T levels among men with ED. **ED and low T are markers of poor health which impact on an individual's self-perception of their health status** (Brooke, et al., 2014).

The Relationship between Libido and Testosterone Levels in Aging Men.

Reduced libido is widely considered the most prominent symptomatic reflection of low testosterone levels in men.
   1,632 men aged 40-70 years old at baseline, with follow-up on 922 (56%) at 9 years and 623 (38%) at 15 years. Libido and T displayed a significant association. The difference in mean T levels between those subjects with low libido and those without was small. Low libido exhibits modest positive predictive value in predicting low T. Recent studies have suggested that the effects of T supplementation on sexual function and desire may be

modest and diminish over time. **The role of endogenous T in modulating libido is complex and that an individual's report of low libido should not necessarily be interpreted as evidence of low serum T** (Travison, Morley, Araujo, O'Donnel, & McKinlay, 2006).

Determined Free Serum Testosterone is Better than Total Testosterone as a Predictor of Prostate Cancer Risk.

Total testosterone and free testosterone levels were drawn in 3,364 consecutive men scheduled for a transrectal ultrasound guided prostate biopsy between 2007-2014. The criteria for prostate biopsy were an abnormal digital rectal examination (DRE) and/or a serum PSA level of >4.0 ng/dl. The median age was 68 years old, rate of abnormal DRE 20.3%, and the median PSA was 7.0. The overall prostate cancer detection rate was 38%.

Low serum levels of total testosterone and free testosterone were significantly associated with prostate cancer risk.

Total serum PSA and DRE were significant independent predictors of cancer.

The present study suggested that free testosterone levels better correlated with prostate cancer detection than total testosterone levels. It did not confirm that low testosterone levels increase tumor aggressiveness which has been shown in many other studies (Regis, et al., 2015).

Levels/logistics of testosterone

TESTOSTERONE LEVELS ARE MOST ACCURATE in the morning. It is the standard of care clinically and in research to do levels in the morning typically by 8am. Testosterone can be given several ways. The safest are intramuscular, subcutaneous, topical, or as slow release pellets placed under the skin surgically.

Variability in total testosterone levels in ageing men with symptoms of androgen deficiency.

96 men aged 62.7 +/- 6.8 years old with symptoms of androgen deficiency had total testosterone levels measured on four occasions in a 12-month period. The men were healthy, non-obese men. A single total testosterone level is a reliable predictor of repeat measures taken within a 12-month period. Nevertheless, **with specific cut-off numbers defining hypogonadism, it is reasonable to repeat the level. Using an average of two baseline T values provides good reliability.** Men with normal baseline T levels are unlikely to have subsequent low T levels recorded (Allan, Strauss, Forbes, Paul, & McLachlan, 2011). Many insurance companies mandate a second

low T level before approving testosterone replacement therapy.

A study of middle-aged and older men with benign prostate disease described that a single testosterone level shows excellent correlation with the mean of seven samples taken over a 48-week period. (Vermeulen & Verdonck, 1992)

Hypogonadal prevalence may be as high as 40% in populations of patients with type 2 diabetes (Hackett, et al., 2009).

Effects of Aromatase Inhibition in Elderly Men with Low or Borderline-Low Serum Testosterone Levels.

37 elderly men (aged 62-74 years old) with T levels below 350 ng/dl were randomized into 3 groups for 12 weeks. Anastrozole (Arimidex) is an aromatase inhibitor used to decrease estradiol levels in women with breast cancer. **It has been used off-label for years to increase T levels or diminish T conversion to estrogen therefore decreasing gynecomastia in men taking testosterone.**

Group 1- anastrozole 1 mg daily.
Group 2- anastrozole 1 mg twice weekly.
Group 3- placebo.

Anastrozole's effect on androgen production is likely directly mediated by the reduction in estrogen production. By reducing estradiol synthesis, anastrozole may be a novel way of normalizing low T in older men. Because estradiol is a crucial mediator of hormonal feedback at the pituitary and hypothalamus in men, aromatase inhibition would be expected to promote pituitary stimulation of testicular testosterone production in men. The criticism with anastrozole is that it may not be adequate if the hypothalamic-pituitary-testicular axis is poorly functioning. The hypothalamic-pituitary axis must be at least partially working to get best results. **Anastrozole may be more useful as an adjunct to T therapy. The downside is by reducing estradiol, anastrozole may have a detrimental effect on bone.**

	Bioavailable T (nl 70-320)	Estradiol (nl 10-50)	LH (nl 1.8-8.6)	Total T (nl 270-1070)
Group 1	99 to 207	26 to 17	5.1 to 7.9	343 To 572
Group 2	115 to 178	27 to 8	4.1 to 7.2	397 to 520

Aromatase inhibition increases bioavailable and total T to more youthful normal levels in older men with mild hypogonadism. It is an effective means of increasing T production. Serum estradiol levels are reduced but generally remain within the normal range for men (Leder, Rohrer, Rubin, Gallo, & Longcope, 2004).

The Salivary Testosterone and Cortisol Response to Three Loading Schemes.

Saliva is developing greater acceptance as a medium for steroid hormone determinations. Salivary hormones accurately reflect the free (unbound) hormone in the blood and are of comparable concentration.

If free hormone activity following resistance exercise contributes to protein metabolism during recovery, then load volume (total amount of weight lifted) maybe the most important workout variable to consider when designing workouts to activate the endocrine system and stimulate muscle growth. A workout volume threshold may need to be reached to maximally activate an anabolic environment (Crewther, Cronin, Keogh, & Cook, 2008).

The Effect of Diurnal Variation on Clinical measurement of Serum Testosterone and Other Sex Hormone Levels in Men.

Testosterone levels peak between 0530 and 0800 hours, depending on the study, with trough levels occurring approximately 12 hours later. In men 30-40 years old, testosterone levels were 20-25% lower at 1600 hours than at 0800 hours. **Total T, free T and bioavailable T were on average 30-35% higher in the morning than levels measured in the mid to late afternoon**. The difference declined with age, with a 10% difference at 70 years. The amplitude of diurnal variation of bioavailable T also declined with age. The amplitude of diurnal variation of DHT, FSH, LH, E2, and SHBG at all ages was either considerably smaller or not detectable. **These results support restricting blood sampling to the morning hours for testosterone**. Results indicated that half of the men with at least one of three T measurements less than 300 ng/dl in the afternoon had normal T levels in all three of their assessments in the morning. **These findings support recommendations for performing more than one T measurement to diagnose hypogonadism**. The results of this study do not necessarily apply to patients on T replacement for whom clinicians are making dose adjustments (Brambilla, Matsumoto, Araujo, & McKinlay, 2009).

The Effects of Serum Testosterone, Estradiol, and Sex Hormone Binding Globulin Levels on Fracture Risk in Older Men.

Study examined associations between nonvertebral fracture risk and bioavailable estradiol, bioavailable testosterone, and SHBG over a four-year period. High SHBG has been independently associated with fracture risk. By binding to testosterone and estradiol, SHBG reduces circulating sex steroid concentrations and thereby their cellular actions (LeBlanc, et al., 2009).

The Osteoporotic Fractures in Men Study (MrOS) was conducted in a prospective US cohort in 5,995 community-dwelling men 65 years old or older.

Older men with low bioavailable estradiol or high SHBG levels are at increased risk of nonvertebral fracture. Low bio-estradiol was independently associated with increased fracture risk extends earlier reports of estrogen's importance for men's skeletal health. Remember, some of testosterone is converted to estradiol which promotes better bone health. A nonlinear association between estradiol and fracture risk was noted supporting the hypothesis that a threshold range of bio-estradiol is necessary for skeletal health. A linear relationship would indicate straightforward predictability. When SHBG levels are high, men with low bio T levels have higher risk. SHBG may be a marker for non-skeletal factors affecting fracture risk. SHBG increases with age and decreases with obesity consistent with common clinical findings. **Because bio-estradiol may have a threshold level, estradiol and SHBG levels have clinical** relevance in assessing fracture risk. **Along with checking calcium, phosphorus, intact PTH, vitamin D levels, it may be helpful at times to check SHBG, testosterone and estradiol levels** when assessing osteoporosis risk. (Vandenput, et al., 2017)

One of the key articles in my research brings to light the additional research needed to better answer the question regarding topical testosterone usage.

Injection of testosterone may be safer and more effective than transdermal administration for combating loss of muscle and bone in older men

The most common modes of T administration are patch and gel preparations and IM injection of long-acting T esters. Administered T may be converted to estradiol via the action of aromatase or to dihydrotestosterone (DHT) by the action of 5α-reductase, both of which exert biological actions at estrogen and androgen receptors, respectively. As such, T may be considered both a hormone (because it binds to androgen receptors) and a prohormone for the synthesis of estradiol and DHT. Our recent meta-analysis showed that Transdermal T (patch and gel) elevated serum DHT 5.46-fold, whereas IM-injected T elevates serum DHT only 2.2-fold. This occurs despite the fact that transdermal and IM TRT elevated T to a similar degree and may be explained by higher concentration of 5α-reductase in skin vs. skeletal muscle.

Studies indicate that TRT done by injection repeatedly show better results in regards to increasing muscle mass and maximum strength judged by one maximum repetition of leg strength in a dose dependent fashion.

In older men, low T is associated with osteopenia and increased fracture risk. T administration increases bone mineral density (BMD), mainly by suppressing bone resorption. Estrogens play a more important role in men and women than testosterone for bone strength. TRT may increase BMD in men by a direct effect of T or by an indirect action by conversion to estradiol. Low estradiol is more strongly associated with osteopenia in older men than low T. **Whereas bone protection in response to replacement doses of T requires aromatization, bone protection resulting from high doses of androgen does not appear to.**

In older men, T increases BMD in regions that have a large component of cancellous bone, such as the lumbar spine and hip. These increases are important because they occur at sites where fractures frequently occur in the elderly. Several studies have shown that IM or SQ testosterone have improved bone density in the single digits after a year whereas transdermal testosterone has not. Large clinical trials needed to assess fracture risk following TRT have not yet been conducted.

T may cause edema, breast tenderness, and gynecomastia, effects that are thought to result from elevation of estradiol subsequent to TRT.

Oral TRT produces significant risk for cardiovascular adverse events (RR = 2.20, P = 0.015). Transdermal (patch or gel) TRT produces a nonsignificant directional trend toward CV risk (RR = 1.27), and IM TRT produces a nonsignificant directional trend toward CV protection

(RR = 0.66). Transdermal and oral TRT cause greater elevation of serum DHT (but not T) compared with injected TRT. Serum DHT concentrations following transdermal and oral TRT correspond to the concentrations that have been linked to CV disease and mortality in observational studies. Finasteride (Proscar), inhibitor of 5 alpha reductase type II, and dutasteride (Avodart), inhibitor of 5 alpha reductase types I and II, blocks conversion of T to DHT without interfering in increasing muscle mass or strength.

The higher circulating DHT levels, obtained with transdermal as opposed to injected T, may be responsible for the trend for increased CV risk with transdermal TRT. In observational studies, Shores et al. have shown high DHT is associated with increased cardiovascular events and increased incident ischemic stroke. Zwadlo et al. have shown that cardiac expression of 5α-reductase is markedly increased in humans with heart failure.

Summary and Recommendations

For treatment of older hypogonadal men, there are advantages to administering TRT by injection rather than transdermally or orally. Intramuscular TRT may not pose the same CV risks as transdermal TRT. A possible explanation is that transdermal T causes greater elevation of serum DHT, due to significant expression of 5α-reductase in skin, but not in muscle. In addition, several studies demonstrate that in older hypogonadal men the combination of IM T plus finasteride produces musculoskeletal benefits without the prostate enlargement that results from T alone. It appears that IM-injected T plus finasteride may be both the safest and the most effective treatment for older hypogonadal men. (Borst & Yarrow, 2015)

Testosterone, Dihydrotestosterone, and Incident Cardiovascular Disease and Mortality in the Cardiovascular Health Study.

Context:
Low testosterone (T) is associated with prevalent cardiovascular disease (CVD) and mortality. DHT, a more potent androgen, may also be associated with CVD and mortality, but few studies have examined this.

Objective:
The study objective was to examine whether T and DHT are risk factors for incident CVD and mortality.

Design:
In a longitudinal cohort study, we evaluated whether total T, calculated free T (cFT), DHT, and calculated free DHT were associated with incident CVD and mortality in men in the Cardiovascular Health Study (mean age 76, range 66–97 years) who were free of CVD at the time of blood collection.

Main Outcome:
The main outcomes were incident CVD and all-cause mortality.

Results:
Among 1032 men followed for a median of 9 years, 436 incident CVD events and 777 deaths occurred. In models adjusted for cardiovascular risk factors, total T and cFT were not associated with incident CVD or all-cause mortality, whereas DHT and calculated free DHT had curvilinear associations with incident CVD ($P < .002$ and $P = .04$, respectively) and all-cause mortality ($P < .001$ for both).

Conclusions:
In a cohort of elderly men, DHT and calculated free DHT were associated with incident CVD and all-cause mortality. Further studies are needed to confirm these results and to clarify the underlying physiologic mechanisms.

This is one of the first studies to examine the association of DHT with incident CVD and all-cause mortality in elderly men without a previous history of CVD. We found that DHT and calculated free DHT had curvilinear associations with incident CVD and all-cause mortality. The curvilinear associations of DHT with adverse outcomes suggest that there may be an ideal physiological range for DHT. However, the associations found in this study do not establish a causal relationship between DHT and adverse outcomes because this cannot be ascertained from an observational study (Shores, et al., 2014).

Testosterone and Dihydrotestosterone and Incident Ischemic Stroke in Men in the Cardiovascular Health Study.

Ischemic stroke is a major cause of morbidity and mortality in elderly men. Our main objective was to examine whether testosterone (T) or dihydrotestosterone (DHT) was associated with incident ischemic stroke in elderly men. This is a clinically relevant question as stroke is the 4th leading cause of death in the United States.
DESIGN: Cohort study.
PARTICIPANTS: Elderly men in the Cardiovascular Health Study who had no history of stroke, heart disease or pros-

tate cancer as of 1994 and were followed until December 2010.

MEASUREMENTS: Ischemic stroke.

RESULTS: Among 1,032 men (mean age 76, range 66-97), followed for a median of 10 years, 114 had an incident ischemic stroke. Total T and free T were not significantly associated with stroke risk, while DHT had a nonlinear association with incident stroke (P = 0·006) in analyses adjusted for stroke risk factors. The lowest risk of stroke was at DHT levels of 50-75 ng/dl, with greater risk of stroke at DHT levels above 75 ng/dl or below 50 ng/dl. (DHT Normal levels 11.2-95.5 ng/dl). Results were unchanged when SHBG was added to the model. Calculated free DHT had an inverse linear association with incident ischemic stroke.

CONCLUSIONS: Dihydrotestosterone had a nonlinear association with stroke risk in which there was an optimal DHT level associated with the lowest stroke risk. Further studies are needed to confirm these results and to clarify whether there is an optimal DHT range associated with the least risk of adverse outcomes in elderly men (Shores, et al., 2014).

Hypogonadism and testosterone replacement therapy in end-stage renal disease (ESRD) and transplant patients.

Low testosterone is a common finding in end-stage renal disease (ESRD) and renal transplant patients. Over half of male renal failure patients demonstrate low or low-normal levels of testosterone-a much higher percentage than the

6-9% of men affected in the general population. The etiology is likely multifactorial and the term "uremic hypogonadism" has been coined to describe the hormonal state associated with kidney disease.

The clinical implications of low testosterone are varied and include associations with mood, anemia, muscle mass and strength, bone mass, and sexual function. The use of testosterone supplementation in particular has dramatically increased in the past few years.

The majority of men with ESRD report some form of sexual dysfunction with some studies reporting >80% of ESRD patients affected. CKD patients were 5 times more likely to be anemic if they had low testosterone levels. There was an inverse association between testosterone levels and erythropoiesis-stimulating agents (ESAs) as well, making testosterone a possible target for patients who are hypo-responsive to ESAs.

Testosterone replacement

It is well known that testosterone replacement leads to improvement of muscle mass and strength and bone density. Improvements in energy, positive feelings, and friendliness along with decreased negative feelings including anger and irritability have been previously shown. Improvements in sexual function have likewise been demonstrated.

Conclusions

Men with ESRD and those who have received a renal transplant are often plagued with hypogonadism. Testosterone replacement therapy has surged in the general population and has been shown in small studies to improve the hormonal parameters of ESRD patients. The effects of

LEVELS/LOGISTICS OF TESTOSTERONE

androgen replacement on sexual dysfunction in ESRD or transplant are controversial but studies suggest variable improvement (Snyder & Shoskes, 2016).

Growth Hormone

A LITTLE HISTORY ABOUT THE discovery of growth hormone shows us how one man can change the lives of thousands of people. Choh Hao Li was born in Canton China in 1913 and moved to University of California at Berkeley in 1938 for his doctorate. He is most famous for discovering human growth hormone in 1955 along with luteinizing hormone, follicle-stimulating hormone, and adrenocorticotrophic hormone. One of his last major accomplishments was the discovery of beta-endorphin. At the peak of his growth hormone deficiency program for short-stature children in 1973, 82,500 pituitary glands had been collected to treat about 3,000 children. Cadaver-derived pituitary growth hormone was replaced by recombinant DNA-produced human growth hormone in the 1980s. (Cadaver-derived pituitary growth hormone was implicated in several cases of Creutzfeldt-Jacob disease). Dr. Li was the author or co-author of more than 1,100 scientific articles and received more than 25 scientific awards. He was awarded honorary degrees by 10 universities around the world. What a great man. (Thomas H Maugh II, dec 2, 1987, Times Science Writer and UPI archives).

The FDA has approved Human Growth Hormone (HGH) for the following conditions. (FDA Import Alert 66-71 04/18/2017).

GROWTH HORMONE

1. Hormonal deficiency that causes short stature in children
2. Long-term treatment of growth failure due to lack of GH secretion
3. Long-term treatment of short stature associated with turner syndrome
4. Adult short bowel syndrome
5. Adult deficiency due to rare pituitary tumors or their treatment of.
6. Muscle-wasting disease associated with HIV/AIDS.

The cost of approved HGH is high, averaging several hundred dollars per dose. Because of this high cost, HGH drugs have been counterfeited and unapproved HGH products are offered for sale to U.S. consumers. Performance-enhancing drugs (PEDs) like HGH have been used for decades to reduce body fat and increase skeletal muscle mass. HGH and analogues are sold on the internet, Men's Clinics, Anti-aging Clinics on a regular basis with the main criteria being a good credit card. Various oral preparations (sprays and pills) supposedly containing HGH are also marketed and distributed. HGH is only available in the injectable form. The HGH molecule is too large for absorption across the lining of the oral mucosa and the hormone is digested by the stomach before absorption can occur if taken orally.

HGH is administered by IM or SQ shot. The half-life is only 20-30 minutes, while its biological half-life is much longer at 9-17 hours due to indirect effects. It is a schedule III drug in the same schedule as anabolic steroids. Internet pharmacies are often partnered with a physician willing to write prescriptions for a fee without a physical examination. The 1990 Anabolic Steroids Control Act states "the distribution and possession, with the intent to distribute, of HGH for any use other than the treatment of a disease or other recognized medical condition is a five-year felony under the penalties chapter of the Food, Drug, and Cosmetics Act of the FDA. Many anti-aging clinics use analogs of HGH to protect themselves from criminal prosecution.

    I do think HGH can have additional benefits but dosing and expectations are key ideas. HGH was approved as a drug by the FDA and therefore cannot be marketed as a dietary supplement. I do not have prescribing experience with HGH but the impression I have from the articles is when it is used off-label the dosing is too high causing many side effects. If I wanted to use it off-label, I would want small improvements over several years. For example, muscle mass is lost about 1% per year and we gain about 1 lb. per year and probably gain a little more than 1% fat mass per year. If we take HGH at low doses for 5 years and improve our muscle mass by 1% per year then after 5 years, we would have changed our muscle mass by 10%. Of course, this is all speculation with no hard data to support this let alone the thousands of dollars it costs. Also, it is illegal at this time. (I'm sorry officer, I just did not know it was illegal).

    I am thinking of opening up the first organic anti-aging clinic for both men and women with a complete guarantee associated with every prescription. Patients can line up outside my office and I promise each and every office visit will only last 5 minutes and cost only $25. I will have a clinic on more corners then Starbucks and after 2 years offer a public offering on the stock market and sell for a billion dollars. I will guarantee elevated Growth Hormone levels and also guarantee feeling happier. My secret will be mass produced scripts prescribing more sleep and more regular exercise since that is a great way that has been well-documented and supported in peer-reviewed medical journals to increase Growth Hormone levels. It will also decrease catabolic hormones and promote more anabolic hormones. Enjoy the articles.

Effects of Human Growth Hormone in Men Over 60 Years Old.

This is the article that promoted great interest in anti-aging use of GH (Growth Hormone). After the age of 30, the secretion of GH by the pituitary gland tends to decline along with muscle mass and an increase in fat mass. Growth hormone secretion can be measured indirectly by measuring the plasma concentration of IGF-1 (insulin-like growth factor 1 or somatomedin C). There is little diurnal variation in the plasma IGF-1 levels, and measurements of it are therefore a convenient indicator of growth hormone secretion. If IGF-1 levels fall below 350 units/liter in older adults, no spontaneous circulating pulses of growth hormone can be detected.

The study involved administering biosynthetic human growth hormone for 6 months to 12 healthy men from 61 to 81 years old and 9 men receiving placebo. All men had IGF-1 levels below 350. The treated men received 0.03 mg/kg GH three times /week. The findings after 6 months in the GH treated group.

1. 8.8% increase in lean body mass.
2. 14.4% decrease in adipose-tissue mass.
3. 1.6% increase in average lumbar vertebral bone density.
4. Skin thickness increased 7.1%
5. No significant change in the bone density of the radius or proximal femur.

Conclusions: diminished secretion of GH is responsible in part for the decrease of lean body mass, the expansion of adipose-tissue mass, and the thinning of the skin that occurs in old age. (Rudman, et al., 1990).

Hormone Replacement Therapy and Physical Function in Healthy Older Men. Time to Talk Hormones?

Improving physical function and mobility in a continuously expanding elderly population is a high priority of medicine today. Muscle mass, strength/power, and maximal exercise capacity are major determinants of physical function, and all decline with aging. This contributes to the incidence of frailty and disability observed in older men. Furthermore, it facilitates the accumulation of body fat and development of insulin resistance. Muscle adaptation to exercise is strongly influenced by anabolic endocrine hormones and local load-sensitive autocrine/paracrine growth factors. GH, IGF-I, and testosterone (T) are directly involved in muscle adaptation to exercise because they promote muscle protein synthesis, whereas T and locally expressed IGF-I have been reported to activate muscle stem cells. Although exercise programs improve physical function, in the long-term most older men fail to comply. The GH/IGF-I axis and T levels decline markedly with aging, whereas accumulating evidence supports their indispensable role in maintaining physical function integrity. Several studies have reported that the administration of T improves lean body mass and maximal voluntary strength in healthy older men. On the other hand, most studies have shown that administration of GH alone failed to improve muscle strength despite amelioration of the detrimental somatic changes of aging. Both GH and T are anabolic agents that promote muscle protein synthesis and hypertrophy but work through separate mechanisms, and the combined administration of GH and T, albeit in only a few studies, has resulted in greater efficacy than either hormone alone. Although it is clear that this combined approach is effective, this review concludes that further studies are needed to assess the long-term efficacy and safety of combined hormone replacement therapy in older men before the medical rationale of prescribing hormone replacement therapy for combating the sarcopenia of aging can be established (Giannoulis, Martin, Nair, Umpleby, & Sonksen, 2012).

Growth Hormone Supplementation in the Elderly.

In the developed world, people older than 80 years are the fasting growing subset of the population. In elderly subjects, the 24-hour integrated GH concentration is equal to levels observed in young patients who have Growth Hormone Deficiency. Several investigators have described a 15% to 70% reduction in GH secretory parameters in men and women older than 60 years. **Modest reductions in skeletal muscle mass with aging do not cause functional impairment and disability: however, when skeletal muscle mass relative to body weight is 30% below the mean of young adults, an increase risk of functional impairment and disability is found.**

The development of sarcopenia in the elderly is not the result of one single change occurring during aging but is a consequence of multisystem changes. It should not be forgotten that the changes observed in the seventh, eighth, ninth, and tenth decades have come about from progressive decline of GH secretion from mid-puberty onward. A review of the current data suggests that GH replacement therapy in GH-deficient adults is safe and does not lead to tumor formation. Patients who have acromegaly with sustained increased IGF-1 levels have no significant increase in site-specific cancer rates. After 7 years of GH treatment in GH-deficient adults, no change in insulin sensitivity was found.

Since the discovery of GH releasing peptides in 1976, several types of GH secretagogues (GHSs) have been developed. Only a few groups have studied the effects of GHSs in the elderly. Overall GHSs were well tolerated and their use was safe. Overall, the use of GH or GHSs represent potential treatment or options for prevention of musculoskeletal impairment associated with aging (Nass, Park, & Thorner,, 2007).

The Growth Hormone/Insulin-Like Growth Factor-1 Axis in Exercise and Sport.

People with too little and too much Growth Hormone suffer from decreased muscle strength and decreased ability to tolerate high level exercise stress when compared to age, gender and height matched people. Replacement doses in deficient individuals and inhibition of Growth Hormone in excess states help these individuals return to relatively normal levels. Treatment for both states prolongs lifespan and lessens morbidity and mortality. Giving

Growth Hormone to normal individuals does not show consistent or significant increases in muscle strength or performance. One would not give thyroid medication to someone euthyroid. Maximal oxygen consumption in GHD (Growth Hormone Deficient) adults has been consistently shown to be reduced by estimates ranging from 17% to 27% compared with values predicted for age, gender, and height. Cuneo et al. demonstrated increases in maximum oxygen consumption, maximal power output, and the lactate threshold after 6 months of GH replacement in GHD subjects. GH replacement increased lactate threshold, demonstrating a reduction in fatigue after GH replacement Both deficient and excess states will develop abnormal echocardiograms if the conditions are not treated.

The onset of exercise leads to a 3-fold increase in the rate of lipolysis and a rapid increase in uptake of FFAs into skeletal muscle whereas GHD patients do not show this beneficial degree of adaptation.

There is strong evidence that GH replacement increases lipolysis, FFA availability, and uptake from the circulation more markedly during exercise compared with resting conditions. LBM (lean body mass) is reduced in GHD adults by approximately 7-8% compared with age and gender matched normal subjects.

In contrast to the protein anabolic effects of GH replacement, which occurs within days to weeks of initiation of treatment, the overall body of evidence suggests that long-term but not short-term GH replacement increases and normalizes muscle strength. We need to think of the long-term benefits using physiological doses rather than supra-physiological doses to best evaluate Growth Hormone usage.

Exercise is the most potent stimulus to GH release. GH starts to increase 10 to 20 min after the onset of exercise, peak either at the end or shortly after exercise, and remain elevated for up to 2 hours after exercise.

The GH response to exercise declines with aging, and it has been demonstrated that even in early middle age (mean age 42 years), the GH response to exhaustive exercise is greatly attenuated compared with younger (mean age 21 years) subjects. The GH response was found to be determined by age and physical fitness but not by body fat, implying that maintenance of physical fitness with increased aging is more important in determining GH release than avoidance of increased adiposity.

Patients with acromegaly represent a useful model to study the chronic effect of GH excess. Acromegaly is characterized by marked abnormalities in protein, carbohydrate metabolism, exaggerated facial structures, enlarged feet and hands, myopathic muscle pathology, etc. The degree of pathology correlates with circulating GH levels. Long-standing acromegaly is also associated with impairment in aerobic exercise capacity and cardiac performance. Oxygen consumption and lactate threshold are reduced in patients with acromegaly, compared with normal subjects, and improve after treatment with octreotide (inhibits GH). Despite the increased size of people with excess Growth Hormone it is very unusual to find a person that reaches the professional sports level. People with excess growth hormone before growth end-plates close develop giantism and ones that have excess after growth plates have closed have acromegaly. One of the most famous individuals with excess growth hormone was Andre the Giant. He had giantism and was 6 feet 3 inches at 12 years old. He was a professional wrestler and actor who was in the great 1987 Rob Reiner film "The Princess Bride" with Billy Crystal and Mandy Patinkin. The movie has many famous quotes but my favorite is "my name is Inigo Montoya, you killed my father, prepare to die.' He died from congestive heart failure at age 46 and weighed 520 lbs. He declined to be treated for acromegaly. Premature death from CHF is very typical.

Although GH abuse by athletics is widespread, there is no evidence of its efficacy. The most plausible mechanisms by which administration of supra-physiological doses of GH could improve exercise performance are through increased muscle mass and strength and through increased fatty acid availability resulting in glycogen sparing and increased endurance.

Berggren et al. (2005) administered supra-physiological GH for 28 days to healthy active normal subjects and found no change in oxygen consumption or maximal power output during cycling.

The effects of administration of GH and testosterone alone and in combination for 6 months to healthy elderly men were studied in a more recent well-powered double-blind placebo-controlled trial (2006). LBM (lean body mass) increased with GH alone, whereas there was an increase in muscle mass and a reduction in total body fat after combined treatment. Oxygen consumption also increased significantly in patients who received combined treatment with those who received placebo and those who received either treatment alone.

The two most promising approaches to detection of GH abuse involve measurement of serum markers of GH action and measurement of the relative proportions in serum of the naturally occurring isoforms of GH.

There is preliminary evidence that GH treatment is useful in improving body composition and exercise performance in elderly subjects particularly when used in association with testosterone. In contrast, there is no evidence that GH improves physical performance in obese subjects (Gibney, Healy, & Sönksen, 2007).

Evaluation and Treatment of Adult Growth Hormone Deficiency: An Endocrine Society Clinical Practice Guideline.

A low IGF-1 level, in the absence of catabolic conditions such as poorly controlled diabetes, liver disease, and oral estrogen therapy, is strong evidence for significant GHD and may be useful in identifying patients who may benefit from treatment and therefore require GH stimulation testing.

We suggest that GH therapy of GH-deficient adults improves several cardiovascular surrogate outcomes, including endothelial function, inflammatory cardiovascular biomarkers, lipoprotein metabolism, carotid intima-media thickness (IMT), and aspects of myocardial function, but tends to increase insulin resistance.

We suggest that GH therapy of GH-deficient adults improves the quality of life of most patients. GH dosing regimens be individualized rather than weight-based and start with low doses and be titrated according to clinical response, side effects, and IGF-1 levels. Patients should be monitored at 1-2 month intervals during dose titration and semiannually thereafter with a clinical assessment and an evaluation for adverse effects, IGF-1 levels, and other parameters for GH response. **GH treatment has been approved since 1996**.

GH treatment has not been approved by the FDA as an anti-aging treatment (Molitch, Clemmons, Malozowski, Merriam, & Vance, 2011).

Systematic Review: The Safety and Efficacy of Growth Hormone in the Healthy Elderly.

The authors included randomized, controlled trials that compared GH therapy with no GH therapy or GH and lifestyle interventions (exercise with or without diet) alone.

31 articles describing 18 unique study populations met the inclusion criteria. A total of 220 participants received GH. Mean age was 69 years old and overweight (mean BMI 28). Initial daily GH dose (mean 14ug/kg) and treatment duration (mean 27 weeks) varied. Results were;

> Fat mass decreased 2.1 kg.
> Lean body mass increased 2.1 kg.
> Weight did not change significantly.
> Total cholesterol decreased but not significantly.
> Bone density, lipids did not change.

Patients treated with GH were significantly more likely to experience soft tissue edema, arthralgias, carpal tunnel syndrome, gynecomastia and were somewhat more likely to experience the onset of diabetes and impaired fasting glucose.

Conclusion: The literature published on random, controlled trials evaluating GH therapy in the healthy elderly is limited. It is associated with small changes in body composition and increased rates of adverse events. GH cannot be recommended as an antiaging therapy (Liu, et al., 2007).

IGF1 as predictor of all-cause mortality and cardiovascular disease in an elderly population.

IGF1 is believed to influence ageing and development of cardiovascular disease through complex mechanisms. Increased mortality and risk of CVD have been observed in patients with GH deficiency as well has excess (acromegaly).

642 patients in Copenhagen, 365 females, 277 males, mean age 68 (range 50-89) years old were evaluated for the development of CHF or first major CV event (nonfatal acute MI, fatal coronary artery disease, unstable angina, CHF, stroke or TIA) after median of 5 years. (range 2-63 months). Hospital discharge diagnoses were used.

103 deaths occurred, 48 females and 55 males. 50% died of CVD, 17% died of cancer and 33% died of other causes.

High values of IGF1 independently predicted all-cause mortality but did not influence the overall incidence of first major CV events.

In normal populations, a high GH-IGF1 activity has been linked to development of cancer and pathological increased IGF1 levels as seen in uncontrolled acromegaly is associated with a substantially reduced lifespan, diabetes and cardiac disease. Low IGF1 levels within the normal range seems also to be harmful and associated with CVD.

There is an intricate relationship between IGF1 signaling and mortality and suggests that high endogenous IGF1 levels might be a risk factor for all-cause mortality. **Our results argue against the suggestion that age-related decline in IGF1 levels is harmful and thus against the use of GH as anti-aging therapy among healthy elderly individuals. The authors concluded that the side effects outweigh beneficial effects mainly due to soft tissue edema, arthralgias, and insulin resistance** (Andreassen, et al., 2009).

Long-term testosterone supplementation augments overnight growth hormone secretion in healthy older men.

Evaluate effect of 26 weeks of low dose Testosterone (100 mg IM every 2 weeks) on nocturnal GH secretory dynamic and AM concentrations of IGF1 and IGFBP-3(Insulin-like growth factor binding protein-3 blocks IGF-1 activity) in 34 healthy older men (65-88 years old) with low-normal T and IGF1 levels.

Aging in healthy men is associated with progressive declines in Total T, free T, GH and IGF1. Beginning in the third decade GH secretion in healthy men is reduced by one-half every 7-12 years: older men typically exhibit a 65-80% reduction in GH secretion compared with young men. Administration of 100 mg IM every 2 weeks increased total T by 33% into the mid-normal range, significantly increased nocturnal 12-hr integrated GH secretion, increased AM IGF1 by 22%, with no significant change in IGFBP-3 levels. Physical fitness is also an important positive predictor of GH secretion (Muniyappa, et al., 2007).

Off-label use of hormones as an antiaging strategy: a review.

If Testosterone is used according to international guidelines and plasma levels do not reach supra-physiological levels, serious adverse effects are rare.

DHEA is a steroid prohormone produced by the adrenal gland and transformed in target tissue through intracrine mechanisms to androgens or estrogens. Plasma DHEA levels decline with age. Studies have shown that low DHEA levels are related to a higher risk for atherosclerosis, heart failure, cardiovascular complications, and overall mortality. Most studies show a very satisfying safety profile for DHEA supplementation. The longest study for DHEA supplementation did not exceed 2 years. No data exist on treatment safety regarding hormone-dependent tumors, cardiovascular risk, or mortality for longer treatments. DHEA has the status of a dietary supplement and is sold OTC in the US. In Europe, it is either forbidden or subject to medical prescription. **Physicians prescribing DHEA should consider and inform their patients of the fact that long-term effects concerning efficiency, but also safety, are still uncertain.**

Studies in healthy elderly have shown a higher risk for adverse effects of GH supplementation, such as carpal tunnel syndrome, gynecomastia, and fluid retention. Concerns have also been put forward about a dose-dependent increase of insulin resistance with GH treatment (Samaras, Papadopoulou, Samaras, & Ongaro, 2014).

Effects of Growth Hormone on Glucose, Lipid, and Protein Metabolism in Human Subjects.

In terms of evolution, the effects of GH are simple: during conditions of excess food, GH in concert with IGF-1 and insulin, promote protein synthesis and storage, and when food is sparse, GH alters fuel consumption from the use of carbohydrates and protein to the use of lipids, thereby allowing conservation of vital protein stores. Our bodies conserve valuable resources to survive. In man, GH is secreted episodically from the pituitary gland with a major surge at the onset of slow-wave sleep and less conspicuous secretory episodes a few hours after meals. A healthy young adult secretes roughly 0.25 mg/m2 body surface of GH per 24 hours (about 0.4-0.5 mg/24 hour). Accumulation of visceral fat rather than chronological age is the most important predictor of GH status in midlife adults. Circulating IGF-1 is predominately stimulated by GH and is produced in the liver in the presence of sufficient nutrient intake and elevated portal insulin levels, and IGF-1 is critical for promoting the protein anabolic effects of GH. The predominant effect of GH is stimulation of lipolysis and lipid oxidation while conserving glucose and protein (counterregulatory stress hormone).

Active acromegaly is associated with glucose intolerance despite compensatory hyperinsulinemia, and hepatic as well as peripheral insulin resistance, and it is likely that these aberrations contribute to the excess mortality. **Insu-**

lin resistance as a side effect to GH administration is no less surprising than the risk of hypoglycemia with insulin therapy. At the present stage, it is important to emphasize that meta-analyses of published data do not justify GH as either an anti-aging treatment or as adjunct treatment in obesity. GH treatment in HIV-associated wasting has been shown in several randomized controlled trials to increase LBM and body weight and to improve physical endurance and quality of life, and GH is a FDA approved indication for this condition (Møller & Jørgensen, 2009).

Growth hormone treatment in human ageing: benefits and risks.

In the few studies designed to evaluate the independent effects of GH treatment and lifestyle interventions (exercise program and resistance training), no significant differences were found in body composition outcomes between subjects treated with GH plus lifestyle intervention and those related with GH alone. Furthermore, these studies could not demonstrate any additional effects of GH on strength training in terms of increased muscle strength, resistance or physical performance. Quite early it was shown that GH administration in healthy elderly individuals very frequently caused acute adverse effects, such as fluid retention, carpal tunnel syndrome and gynecomastia. Increased glucose and insulin concentrations, resulting from differing degrees of insulin resistance, have been recorded during GH therapy in a dose-dependent manner. It has been clearly demonstrated in several animal models that reduced GH and IGF-1 levels or actions are associated with significant increases in both average and maximal lifespan. GH cannot be recommended for use by the healthy elderly, bearing in mind that GH decline with age may represent a beneficial adaptation to ageing. At present, no definitive answers can be provided to the safety of long-term GH or GH-releasing peptide intervention in elderly individuals with the aim of reversing the effects of somatopause (Giordano, Bonelli, Marinazzo, Ghigo, & Arvat, 2008).

Recombinant human growth hormone treatment in elderly patients undergoing elective total hip replacement.

33 patients (23 females, 10 males, aged 60-82 years old) scheduled for hip replacement. Study was double-blind, placebo-controlled with parallel groups. GH or placebo was administered for 14 weeks preoperatively (0.04U/kg/day) and 4 weeks postoperatively (with dose doubled for first two weeks postoperatively).

Lean body mass increased 5.2% preoperatively with GH but fell 3% postoperatively in both groups. Mid-thigh muscle cross-sectional area remained same in GH group but decreased 10% in placebo. There was a trend towards a favorable effect of GH on strength in the majority of muscles tested, but this was significant only for the abductors of the non-operated hip, where there was a 7% increase in strength over the whole study compared with a 25% decrease in the placebo group. Dose-related side effects were seen in the patients receiving GH.

Conclusion-preoperative GH in modest doses to elderly patients awaiting total hip replacement results in improvements in lean body mass and skeletal muscle mass that are sufficient to offset the losses that occur postoperatively (Weissberger, et al., 2003).

What is interesting to me is the rapid loss of muscle strength and lean body mass over such a short period of time emphasizing the importance of improving supportive muscles around joints to preserve longevity and the need to always avoid bedrest if possible. Getting "back on the horse is always good advice."

Effects of Recombinant Human Growth Hormone Therapy in Obesity in Adults: A Meta-analysis.

Endogenous secretion of GH is decreased in obesity. 477 subjects completed the studies with mean age 25.4 to 67.5 years old (median 38 years) and their mean BMI ranged from 28-42 kg/m2. Ten studies included only women, and four studies only men. Treatment duration ranged from 3-72 weeks (median 11.5 weeks).

GH leads to a decrease in total visceral adiposity, an increase in lean body mass, favorable changes in lipid profile but does not affect overall body weight. These effects appear to be quantitatively small and would not justify a clinically relevant role for GH in obesity particularly in view of the supra-physiological GH dose used in many studies as well as the high cost of it. A clear association occurs with dose and presence of arthralgias, edema and paresthesias (Mekala & Tritos, 2009).

Growth Hormone and Sex Steroid Administration in Healthy Aged Women and Men. A Randomized Controlled Trial.

26-week randomized, double-blind, placebo-controlled parallel-group trial in healthy, ambulatory, community-dwelling US women (57) and men (74) aged between 65-88 years old.

Group 1-placebo.
Group 2-GH (30ug/kg, decreased to 20ug/kg SQ 3x/week).
Group 3-HRT (estradiol/medroxyprogesterone for women, T 100 mg IM every 2 weeks for men) HRT- hormone replacement therapy.
Group 4-GH and HRT.

Systolic and diastolic blood pressures and mean pulse rates did not change significantly in any treatment group.

A 6.8% increase in strength in men treated with GH and Testosterone was of marginal statistical significance. An increase in the magnitude observed would be expected typically after 6-8 weeks of regular resistance exercise and is potentially clinically significant. Cardiovascular endurance capacity increased significantly only in men after GH and Testosterone treatment. **The magnitude of the increases in LBM (lean body mass) and decreases in fat following GH and Testosterone treatment were similar to 6 months of exercise training 3 times per week and greater than those observed after training once per week.**

Most but not all previous studies reported no effect of GH on strength in aged individuals, consistent with our findings after GH alone.

Peripheral edema, carpal tunnel symptoms, and arthralgias occurred in 24% of GH-treated participants. Diabetes and glucose intolerance developed significantly more often after GH treatment in men, as others have reported (Blackman, et al., 2002). Several articles express positive benefits when Growth Hormone and testosterone are used together. Lower doses could be used while decreasing side effects of both drugs.

Durability of the effects of testosterone and growth hormone supplementation in older community dwelling men: the HORMA trial.

108 community-dwelling elderly men (71 +/- 4 years old) were placed on transdermal T and recombinant growth hormone therapy for 16 weeks with subsequent evaluation at week 28. **Those who had gains in lean body mass and decreases in fat mass at week 17 had significant retention of favorable changes in body composition persisted at 28 weeks.** This study raises the possibility that if the decline in physical function in the frail elderly can be sufficiently reversed, then the gains in muscle mass and strength may be retained by improved functional capacity, breaking the downward cycle of ever increasing weakness and debility (Sattler, et al., 2011).

Muscle Beach

TESTOSTERONE IS A CONTROLLED DRUG that requires a prescription. In 1970 the FDA released a drug classification/drug schedule system under the Controlled Substance Act. The drug classification organizes drugs into groups based on risk of abuse or harm.

1. Schedule 1 Controlled Substance-no currently accepted medical use in the U.S, high abuse potential and significant safety issues. Examples are heroin, Ecstasy, LSD.
2. Schedule 2 Controlled Substance-high abuse potential. Examples are narcotics, and amphetamines. Some narcotics are hydromorphone (Dilaudid), oxycodone (Oxycontin, Percocet), fentanyl (Duragesic), morphine and codeine. Schedule 2 amphetamines include Adderall, Ritalin. Refills are not allowed on prescriptions. Schedule 2 drugs must be written on a prescription. Only in emergency conditions can it be phoned in followed by a written prescription. Some states are going to electronic prescriptions only and narcotics can only be given as 1 week supplies.
3. Schedule 3 Controlled Substance- moderate to low abuse or dependence. Testosterone and other anabolic steroids. Prescriptions for Schedule 3 and 4 drugs can have refills up to 6 months.
4. Schedule 4 Controlled Substance-low abuse potential such as many anxiety medications such as alprazolam

(Xanax), lorazepam (Ativan), carisoprodol (Soma-muscle relaxer), and phentermine (weight loss medicine). Refills up to 6 months can be given.

Since testosterone is a controlled drug, it needs to be written and supervised by a medical professional with a license to prescribe it. Testosterone and other anabolic steroids can be obtained on the internet and other questionable sources. The concern is obvious. The articles below reveal the dangers of abuse along with the counterproductive habits typically followed. The old idea that if one pill is good then 2 pills must be better starts to describe the mind-set. A more realistic mission statement for users would be- if 2 pills are better than a handful of pills or injections is just right. The usage of essentially similar anabolic steroids together in mind-blowing doses only increases side effects and really decreases potential results. One could easily obtain the same or even better results by using much lower doses and avoiding many combinations of different drugs that increase potential dangers. Most doctors are willing to give non-judgmental advice to bodybuilders and bodybuilders should not be afraid that someone is going to blow the whistle on them.

The Changing Drug Culture: Use and Misuse of Appearance- and Performance-Enhancing Drugs.

Abstract
Awareness of the prevalence of the use of appearance- and performance-enhancing drugs (APEDs) is increasing. Users range from professional athletes and bodybuilders to amateurs and adolescents. Anabolic androgenic steroids (AASs)

are the most widely used APEDs, typically for purposes of building muscle mass, in forms that include pills, injections, topical preparations, and transdermal systems. AASs are often used in combination with augmenting drugs taken to enhance androgen production and, for men, to decrease estrogen production. These include aromatase inhibitors, clomiphene, selective estrogen receptor modulators, and human chorionic gonadotropin. Other drugs used with the intention of improving athletic performance include human growth hormone, insulin-like growth factor 1, insulin, erythropoietin, stimulants, diuretics, levothyroxine, and gamma-hydroxybutyrate. Use of APEDs is increasing, with up to 5% of male and 2% of female college athletes using AASs and reports of a more than 20% usage rate among teenagers. **Although many of these substances can increase muscle mass when combined with high levels of exercise and specific diets, it is not clear that they improve athletic performance.** Furthermore, they are associated with a variety of serious adverse effects. AASs, in particular, can cause hepatotoxicity and acute cardiac events. Behavioral and psychiatric symptoms also can occur (Albertson, Chenoweth, Colby, & Sutter, 2016).

MECHANISMS IN ENDOCRINOLOGY: Medical consequences of doping with anabolic androgenic steroids: effects on reproductive functions.

Abstract

The global lifetime prevalence of AASs abuse is 6.4% for males and 1.6% for women. Many AASs, have not undergone proper testing and are consumed at extremely high doses and in irrational combinations, also along with other drugs. Controlled clinical trials investigating undesired side effects are lacking because ethical restrictions prevent exposing volunteers to potentially toxic regimens, obscuring a causal relationship between AASs abuse and possible sequelae. Because of the negative feedback in the regulation of the hypothalamic-pituitary-gonadal axis, in men AASs cause reversible suppression of spermatogenesis, testicular atrophy, infertility, and erectile dysfunction (anabolic steroid-induced hypogonadism). Should spermatogenesis not recover after AASs abuse, a pre-existing fertility disorder may have resurfaced. AASs frequently cause gynecomastia and acne. In women, AASs may disrupt ovarian function. Chronic strenuous physical activity leads to menstrual irregularities and, in severe cases, to the female athlete triad (low energy intake, menstrual disorders and low bone mass), making it difficult to disentangle the effects of sports and AASs. Acne, hirsutism and (irreversible) deepening of the voice are further consequences of AASs misuse. There is no evidence that AASs cause breast carcinoma. Detecting AASs misuse through the control network of the World Anti-Doping Agency (WADA) not only aims to guarantee fair conditions for athletes, but also to protect them from medical sequelae of AASs abuse (Nieschlag & Vorona, 2015).

Natural bodybuilding competition preparation and recovery: a 12-month case study.

Abstract
Bodybuilding is a sport in which competitors are judged on muscular appearance. This case study tracked a drug-

free male bodybuilder (age 26-27 y) for 6 months before and after a competition.

PURPOSE:

The aim of this study was to provide the most comprehensive physiological profile of bodybuilding competition preparation and recovery ever compiled.

METHODS:

Cardiovascular parameters, body composition, strength, aerobic capacity, critical power, mood state, resting energy expenditure, and hormonal and other blood parameters were evaluated.

RESULTS:

Heart rate decreased from 53 to 27 beats/min during preparation and increased to 46 beats/min within 1 month after competition. Brachial blood pressure dropped from 132/69 to 104/56 mmHg during preparation and returned to 116/64 mmHg at 6 months after competition. Percent body fat declined from 14.8% to 4.5% during preparation and returned to 14.6% during recovery. Strength decreased during preparation and did not fully recover during 6 months of recovery. Testosterone declined from 9.22 to 2.27 ng/mL during preparation and returned to the baseline level, 9.91 ng/mL, after competition. Total mood disturbance increased from 6 to 43 units during preparation and recovered to 4 units 6 months after competition.

CONCLUSIONS:

This case study provides a thorough documentation of the physiological changes that occurred during natural bodybuilding competition and recovery (Rossow, Fukuda, Fahs, Loenneke, & Stout, 2013).

It is impressive what someone can do without drugs and also how are body returns to prior steady state. Heavy exercise decreases testosterone levels.

Effects of heavy-resistance training on hormonal response patterns in younger vs. older men.

Two groups of men (30 and 62 yr. old) participated in a 10-wk strength-power training program. Heavy-resistance exercise has been shown to be a potent stimulus for acute increases in circulating hormones in younger men. In contrast, heavy-resistance exercise has not been shown to elicit the same magnitude of hormonal responses in older men. The following study looked at this. Training the older group demonstrated a significant increase in total testosterone in response to exercise stress along with significant decreases in resting cortisol. Older men do respond with an enhanced hormonal profile in the early phase of a resistance training program, but the response is different from that of younger men. Restoring an endocrine gland's function with exercise training remains an attractive hypothesis, which could help ameliorate the age-related declines in muscle tissue mass and strength. The other primary finding was the endocrine system demonstrated a "plasticity" for adaptational changes in older and younger men in the early phase of a heavy-resistance training program. The exercised induced concentrations of testosterone were significantly higher in the 30 years old group compared to the 62 years old group.

30 years-old (after 10-wk training) total T 585 ng/dl, and free T 80

62 years-old (after 10-wk training) total T 452 ng/dl, and free T 60

The amount of cortisol produced at resting levels was reduced with training but the response to resistance exercise was lower in older men. **Older men can reduce the catabolic hormonal response by exercising resulting in a more favorable anabolic environment for reduced protein degradation and increased protein synthesis** (Kraemer, et al., 1999).

Effect of Moderate to Vigorous Physical Activity on All-Cause Mortality in Middle-aged and Older Australians.

Prospective cohort study looking at all-cause mortality in 204,542 adults aged 45 through 75 years over an 8-year period looking at death rate and amount of moderate to vigorous exercise activity.

1. Low time 10-149 minutes/week. Death rate 4.81%
2. Moderate time 150-299 minutes/week. Death rate 3.17%
3. Large time 300 minutes/week or more. Death rate 2.64%

There was an inverse dose-response relationship between proportion of vigorous activity and mortality (Gebel, et al., 2015).

High-resistance weight training produces greater improvement in muscle strength than pharmacological intervention but usually requires three sessions per week of intense exercise over several months.

Synchronous deficits in cumulative muscle protein synthesis and ribosomal biogenesis underlie age-related anabolic resistance to exercise in humans

Twenty healthy males, 10 young (23 +/- 1year) and 10 older (69 +/- 3 years), performed 6 weeks of UNILATERAL resistance exercise training. Bilateral muscle biopsies were performed to look at protein synthesis/muscle hypertrophy response to UNILATERAL exercise only. Muscle mass is controlled by the diurnal balance between muscle protein synthesis and protein breakdown.

Key points;

1. Resistance exercise training (RET) is one of the most effective strategies for preventing declines in skeletal muscle mass and strength with age.
2. Hypertrophic responses to RET with age are diminished compared to younger individuals.
3. In response to 6 weeks RET, we found blunted hypertrophic responses with age are underpinned by chronic deficits in long-term muscle protein synthesis.
4. We show this is likely to be the result of multifactorial deficits in anabolic hormones and anabolic systems.

(Brook, et al., 2016)

The effects of supra-physiological doses of testosterone on angry behavior in healthy eugonadal men-a clinical research center study.

Anecdotal reports of "roid rage" and violent crimes by androgenic steroid users have brought attention to the relationship between anabolic steroid use and angry outbursts. 43 eugonadal men, age 19-40 years old were randomized to 1 of 4 groups in a double-blind, placebo-controlled design. Competitive athletes, and individuals with psychiatric disorders were excluded. **600 mg testosterone enanthate IM per week for ten weeks were given. (typical replacement dose 75-125 mg/week).**

Group 1-placebo, no exercise
Group 2-testosterone, no exercise
Group 3-placebo, exercise
Group 4-testosterone plus exercise

Exercise consisted of three times per week. To assess anger each participant and his significant other were given questionnaires measuring different aspects of anger. The questionnaires were the Multi-Dimensional Anger Inventory (MAI), Mood Inventory(MI), to the participant and the Observer Mood Inventory(OMI) to his significant other (spouse, live-in partner, or parent). No differences were observed in any of the groups to mood or outward behavior.

It would have been nice if questionnaires were given both before and after T treatment. A criticism is 10 weeks does not predict future behavior. The dose used is several times the recommended dose yet many bodybuilders will use even higher doses. Safety and ethical issues appropriately limited the dose. It does show that doses much higher than replacement doses are safe to give to young healthy men. Many scientific and non-scientific reports seem to show aggression may occur at very high supraphysiological doses that unfortunately are used routinely by some athletes (Tricker, et al., 1996).

Heavy Testosterone Use Among Bodybuilders. An Uncommon Cohort of Illicit Substance Users.

An anonymous, self-administered, 49-item questionnaire was posted on message boards of Internet websites popular among AAS (androgenic-anabolic steroids) users.

231 male respondents met criteria.

92.6 % used substances in addition to testosterone.

87% used antiestrogen agents.

86% reported subjective adverse effects with testosterone use. Testicular atrophy, acne, and fluid retention most common.

86.4% experienced subjective adverse effects when not taking testosterone. (addiction dilemma and withdrawal).

81% use 400 mg testosterone or more per week (usual medical dose is about 75-125 mg/week).

16.5% used more than 1000 mg testosterone per week.

77.1% have routine lab tests. Of those having lab tests 38% had lab abnormalities.

69.2 % regularly see a physician.

56% never have informed personal physician of AAS use.

57.6 % were between 18-34 years old.

83.1% completed at least some college.

53% had taken illegal drugs.

47.6% earned 75,000 or more pre-tax.

61.9% played high school sports.

39% used testosterone from 1-3 years.

15.6% played collegiate sports.

52.7% used the Internet for obtaining Testosterone.

27.9% received Testosterone from a physician.

19% used overseas supplier.

9.3% reported personally knowing someone who had been directly harmed by testosterone use.

7.1% used anti-aging clinic.

(Westerman, et al., 2016)

Prolonged Hypogonadism in Males Following Withdrawal from Anabolic-Androgenic Steroids: an Underrecognized Problem.

To assess the frequency and severity of hypogonadal symptoms in male long-term anabolic-androgenic steroid (AAS) misusers who have discontinued AAS use.

INTRODUCTION

Early studies of AAS users have generally suggested that hypogonadism will gradually resolve after AAS use is discontinued. At least eight reports describe cases of hypogonadism and/or azoospermia persisting more than a year after last AAS use.

Discussion

Findings suggest that these symptoms may persist for more than a year after the last AAS use, and possibly much longer.

Hypogonadal symptoms may induce individuals to quickly resume AAS use after stopping a prior course of these drugs, in an attempt to self-treat dysphoric sexual and mood symptoms. Repeated cycles of AAS re-use may then lead to AAS dependence, a disorder that appears to develop in as many as 30% of illicit AAS users.

Conclusions

Among long-term anabolic-androgenic steroid misusers, anabolic-androgenic steroid-withdrawal hypogonadism appears to be common, frequently prolonged, and associated with substantial morbidity.

In contrast to other drugs of abuse high dose testosterone is largely an adult phenomenon. Only 22% of users began using testosterone before the age of 20 years (Kanayama, et al., 2015).

Psychiatric and medical effects of anabolic-androgenic steroid use. A controlled study of 160 athletes.

88 athletes using steroids with 68 nonusers, using the Structured Clinical Interview for DSM-III-R to diagnose psychiatric syndromes with steroid use (if applicable) and in the absence of steroid use. Demographic, medical, and laboratory measures were also performed.

Steroid users displayed more frequent gynecomastia, decreased mean testicular length, and higher cholesterol/HDL ratios than nonusers. Most strikingly, 23% of steroid users reported major mood syndromes--mania, hypomania, or major depression--in association with steroid use. Steroid users displayed mood disorders during steroid exposure significantly more frequently than in the absence of steroid exposure ($P < .001$) and significantly more frequently than nonusers ($P < .01$). Users rarely abused other drugs simultaneously with steroids.

CONCLUSION:

Major mood disturbances associated with anabolic-androgenic steroids may represent an important public health problem for athletes using steroids and sometimes for the victims of their irritability and aggression (Pope & Katz, 1994).

I chose this article to emphasize that the negative effects of anabolic-androgenic steroid use have been known for decades. This study is 23 years old. What has evolved or worsened is that steroid users now use polypharmacy routines to bulk up instead of only one agent. Remember, in 1994, there were 4,000 supplements, and in 2012, more than 80,000 supplements are available. I suspect the doses used now are much higher and the number of different drugs used in combinations are also a lot higher.

Nutrition, Pharmacological and Training Strategies Adopted by Six Bodybuilders: Case Report and Critical Review.

The purpose of this study was to report and analyze the practices adopted by bodybuilders in light of scientific evidence and to propose evidence-based alternatives. Six (four male and two female) bodybuilders and their coaches were directly interviewed. According to the reports, the quantity of anabolic steroids used by the men was 500–750 mg/week during the bulking phase and 720–1160 mg during the cutting phase. The values for women were 400 and 740 mg, respectively. The participants also used ephedrine and hydrochlorothiazide during the cutting phase. Resistance training was designed to train each muscle once per week and all participants performed aerobic exercise in the fasted state in order to reduce body fat. During the bulking phase, bodybuilders ingested ~2.5

g of protein/kg of body weight. (typical medical guideline is 0.8 -1.5 grams protein/kg). During the cutting phase, protein ingestion increased to ~3 g/kg and carbohydrate ingestion decreased by 10–20%. During all phases, fat ingestion corresponded to ~15% of the calories ingested. The supplements used were whey protein, chromium picolinate, omega 3 fatty acids, branched chain amino acids, poly-vitamins, glutamine and caffeine. The men also used creatine in the bulking phase. In general, the participants gained large amounts of fat-free mass during the bulking phase; however, much of that fat-free mass was lost during the cutting phase along with fat mass. Based on our analysis, we recommend an evidence-based approach by people involved in bodybuilding, with the adoption of a more balanced and less artificial diet. One important alert should be given for the combined use of anabolic steroids and stimulants, since both are independently associated with serious cardiovascular events. A special focus should be given to revisiting resistance training and avoiding fasted cardio in order to decrease the reliance on drugs and thus preserve bodybuilders' health and integrity (Gentil, et al., 2017).

I used to be a 98 lb wrestler in high school and I can personally state that exercising in a fasted or very low-calorie state is absolutely not fun.

Anabolic steroids, acute myocardial infarction and polycythemia: A case report and review of the literature

The association between testosterone-replacement therapy and cardiovascular risk remains unclear with most reports suggesting a neutral or possibly beneficial effect of the hormone in men and women. However, several cardiovascular complications including hypertension, cardiomyopathy, stroke, pulmonary embolism, fatal and nonfatal arrhythmias, and myocardial infarction have been reported with supraphysiologic doses of anabolic steroids. We report a case of an acute ST-segment elevation myocardial infarction in a patient with traditional cardiac risk factors (tobacco, family history) using supraphysiologic doses of supplemental, intramuscular testosterone. In addition, this patient also had polycythemia, likely secondary to high-dose testosterone. The patient underwent successful percutaneous intervention of the right coronary artery. Phlebotomy was used to treat the polycythemia acutely. We suggest that the chronic and recent "stacked" use of intramuscular testosterone as well as the resultant polycythemia and likely increased plasma viscosity may have been contributing factors to this cardiovascular event, in addition to traditional coronary risk factors. Physicians and patients should be aware of the clinical consequences of anabolic steroid abuse (Stergiopoulos, Brennan, Mathews, Setaro, & Kort, 2008).

Acute myocardial infarction in a young bodybuilder taking anabolic androgenic steroids: A case report and critical review of the literature.

Abstract
We describe a case report of a 30-year-old bodybuilder suffering an acute myocardial infarction (AMI). He had been taking stanozolol and testosterone for two months.

The coronary angiogram showed high thrombotic burden in the left anterior descending artery without underlying atherosclerosis. Few case reports of AMI in athletes taking anabolic androgenic steroids (AASs) have been reported so far. AAS-related AMI is possibly underreported in the medical literature due to the desire of the affected individuals to hide AAS use. Physicians should always consider the possibility of AAS abuse in the context of a young athlete suffering AMI. AASs can predispose to AMI through the acceleration of coronary atherosclerosis. Additionally, thrombosis without underlying atherosclerosis or vasospasm is highly possible to cause AMI in AAS users. Complications after AMI may be more frequent in AAS users (Christou G. , Christou, Nikas, & Goudevenos, 2016).

If anyone reading this book is not in the medical field one needs to appreciate that the left anterior descending coronary artery has the dubious label as the "widow-maker" signifying the potential poor prognosis without rapid intervention. This is serious business.

Adverse Health Consequences of Performance-Enhancing Drugs: An Endocrine Society Scientific Statement.

Androgenic-anabolic steroids are the most frequently used class of Performance Enhancing Drugs (PEDs).

Because widespread illicit PED use did not appear in the general population until the 1980s and 1990s, the great majority of world's PED users are still under the age of 50 today. As such, this relatively young population has not reached the age of risk for a range of diseases, such as cardiovascular problems, that typically arise later in life. This likely explains why, to date, only occasional case reports have highlighted acute medical events and deaths associated with PEDs. And it's likely that some of the long-term effects of PEDs will only start to become visible as the older members of the PED-using population reach the age of risk for these phenomena. Therefore, **current observations likely underestimate the full magnitude of medical consequences of PEDs that will become evident over the next 2 or 3 decades.**

- Some 2% of American high school students report used androgenic-anabolic steroids (AAS) in the past 12 months.
- The median age of usage of PEDs across all studies consistently fell into the narrow range of 22 to 24 years.
- 2.9-4.0 Americans are estimated to have used an androgenic-anabolic steroid (AAS) at some time.
- 32.5% of AAS users develop AAS dependence.

Androgenic-anabolic steroids (AAS) may induce effects on the brain reward system that may render individuals susceptible to other drugs of abuse and PED users often use other drugs both legal and illegal. High-risk health behaviors are not uncommon.

AAS abusers have been found to develop many cardiac effects. They include left ventricular hypertrophy, cardiac fibrosis, ventricular repolarization abnormalities, decreased ejection fraction, decreased HDL cholesterol, elevated LDL cholesterol, and increased coronary artery calcium scores. Psychiatric effects are higher in AAS users and depend greatly on the doses used. **Mood disorders are greatly increased when users are using more than**

1000 mg testosterone per week (standard dose is 75-125 mg every week). The AAS-induced aggression is sufficiently established that it likely meets the American standard for admissibility as legal testimony.

There is little evidence that hGH (human growth hormone) in supra-physiological doses affects physical performance. A systematic review of randomized trials concluded that although hGH increases lean body mass, it may not improve strength. The scientific literature does not support claims that hGH administration enhances physical performance, but there is some evidence regarding the effects of hGH on some athletic performance outcomes, such as anaerobic capacity. Lance Armstrong is a good example. Adverse effects include edema, excessive sweating, myalgias, arthralgias, carpal tunnel syndrome, and diabetes (Pope, et al., 2014).

Heavy Resistance Training and Supplementation with the Alleged Testosterone Booster NMDA Has No Effect on Body Composition, Muscle Performance, and Serum Hormones Associated with the Hypothalamus-Pituitary-Gonadal Axis in Resistance-Trained Males.

NMDA is a supplement sold that advertises significant increases in testosterone causing greater performance not only in the gym but also in the bedroom. NMDA stands for N-Methyl-D-Aspartic Acid. Like all supplements, the claims are not supported or verified by the FDA.

Twenty resistance-trained males engaged in 28 days of resistance training 4 times/week while orally ingesting either 1.78 grams of placebo or 1.78 grams NMDA

(N-methyl-D-aspartate). Total body mass, fat-free mass and muscle strength were significantly increased in response to resistance training. **All serum hormones (total and free testosterone, LH, GnRH, estradiol, cortisol, prolactin) were unaffected by resistance training or NMDA supplementation** (Willoughby, Spillane, & Schwarz, 2014).

NMDA could stand for Non-Muscle-Development-Again (sarcasm is only effective in minute doses).

Designer steroids-over-the-counter supplements and their androgenic component: review of an increasing problem.

Designer anabolic steroids referred to by various names as pro-hormones, natural steroids, testosterone boosters, have been popular for over a decade to achieve classic anabolic steroid-like results from products sold in the legal marketplace. A "designer steroid" is an anabolic-androgenic steroid synthesized from a known parent steroid and chemically modified with the intent to circumvent controlled substances laws. Recent evidence suggests that anabolic steroid use may be the most common cause of hypogonadism in men of reproductive age. Despite recent regulatory efforts to ban specific compounds, many anabolic-androgenic steroids (AAS) remain available in over-the-counter dietary supplements that are legally sold in the United States. Severe side effects include hepatotoxicity, cholestasis, renal failure, hypogonadism, gynecomastia and infertility.

Since 2002, potent synthetic oral AAS have been detected in as many as 20% of legally sold sports nutrition products. With global sales of dietary supplements reaching tens of billions of dollars yearly, significant public consumption of these over-the-counter AAS can be inferred. A vast number of designer steroids exist, many are novel compounds with no associated published research. **Most designer AAS are analogues of compounds initially developed in the 1960s-early generation synthetic androgens abandoned in the pipeline for better alternatives. Essentially inferior products are abused to avoid detection.** Multiple studies have exposed "nutraceuticals" containing AAS not included on their product label. Chemists may employ methods to deliver potent androgens without technically selling controlled substances by using pro-drugs that are unclassified compounds in the bottle, but in vivo are metabolized to Schedule III controlled AAS.

Currently popular designer steroids are

1. Dimethazine (DMZ)
2. Methylclostebol (German athletes in the 1960s and 1970s used it).
3. Mentabolan
4. Methylepitiostanol (Epistane)
5. Methylstenbolone (Ultradrol)

About 30% of classic AAS users develop dependence, and the ease of availability of designer steroids contribute to a dependence disorder (Rahnema, Crosnoe, & Kim, 2015).

Effects of Anabolic Androgenic Steroids on the Reproductive System of Athletes and Recreational Users: A Systematic Review and Meta-Analysis.

Systematic review and meta-analysis aimed to critically assess the impact of anabolic androgenic steroids (AAS) use on the reproductive system of athletes and recreational users. Thirty-three studies with 3,879 participants with 1,766 AAS users and 2,113 non-AAS users. The majority of the participants were men: only six studies provided data for female athletes. During AAS usage, significant reductions in LH (luteinizing hormone), FSH (follicle-stimulating hormone), and testosterone levels were reported. After AAS discontinuation, serum gonadotropin levels gradually returned to baseline values within 13-24 weeks, whereas serum testosterone levels remained lower as compared with baseline. Serum testosterone levels remained reduced at 16 weeks. AAS abuse resulted in structural and functional sperm changes, a reduction in testicular volume, gynecomastia, as well as clitoramegaly, menstrual irregularities, and subfertility (Christou M. , et al., 2017).

Former Abusers of Anabolic Androgenic Steroids Exhibit Decreased Testosterone levels and Hypogonadal Symptoms Years after Cessation: A Case-Control Study.

The study had a cross-sectional case-control design and involved 37 current AAS abusers, 33 former AAS abusers (elapsed duration 2.5 years (1.7 to 3.7 years) and 30 healthy controls. All participants were aged 18-50 years and were involved in recreational strength training. The total duration of accumulated AAS abuse for current users was 142 weeks (100-203 weeks) was not significantly different from former users 112 weeks (81-154 weeks), and the number of compounds used did not differ between the two groups. The two groups reported previous and current experience with varying doses of numerous AAS compounds of which testosterone esters, trenbolone, nandrolone, stanozol, sustanon and boldenone were the mostly widely used. High proportions of both current and former AAS abusers reported regularly using hCG or aromatase inhibitors following AAS cycles. Eleven former AAS abusers had previously been referred to an endocrine clinic for gynecomastia but none had been treated for gynecomastia, hypogonadism or infertility. Testicular volume differed statistically among the three groups. Current AAS abusers had the smallest testicular volume 12.2 ml compared to 17.4 ml for former AAS abusers followed by 22.2 ml for control participants. Former AAS abusers exhibited significantly lower median total and free testosterone levels than controls. Overall, 27.2% of former AAS abusers exhibited plasma total testosterone levels below the lower reference limit whereas no control participants exhibited testosterone below this limit (statistically significant). Gonadotropins (LH, FSH) were significantly suppressed, and inhibin B and anti-Mullerian hormone (AMH) were significantly decreased in current AAS abusers compared with former AAS abusers and control participants. 57% of current AAS abusers had levels of inhibin B below the level that impairs spermatogenesis. Inhibin B and anti-Mullerian hormones are involved in male fertility. The group of former AAS abusers had higher proportions of participants with depressive symptoms (24.2%), erectile dysfunction (27.3%), and decreased libido (40.1%) than the other groups. **In conclusion, a high proportion of former AAS abusers exhibited biochemical and functional anabolic androgenic steroid-induced hypogonadism (ASIH) several years after AAS cessation.** Current AAS abusers exhibited biochemical abnormalities suggestive of impaired spermatogenesis, which were associated with increasing accumulated duration of AAS abuse. ASIH may become a public health concern with respect to male infertility and hypogonadism (Rasmussen, et al., 2016).

Two Emerging Concepts for Elite Athletes. The Short-Term Effects of Testosterone and Cortisol on the Neuromuscular System and the Dose-Response Training Role of these Endogenous Hormones.

Resistance training provides an effective stimulus for improving the morphological (muscle size) and/or functional (strength, power) qualities of the neuromuscular system in athletic and non-athletes. By measuring hormone levels with different types of workouts, we may be able to decide which type of workouts provide for the best results for a particular athlete and their particular sport (Crewther, Cook, Cardinale, Weatherby, & Lowe).

Sarcopenia (poverty of the flesh)

AS THE POPULATION GETS OLDER, new conditions are defined that become more prevalent and require attempts at intervention to improve them. One condition is sarcopenia. Other words that are similar include frailty, cachexia, failure to thrive and chronically-ill. Although each word has its own definition the general idea is a state of deterioration. **Sarcopenia is the degenerative loss of skeletal muscle mass to the level that it interferes with independence.** A working definition was proposed by Baumgartner et al in 1998 using a dual energy X-ray absorptiometry (DEXA) that defined sarcopenia as having lean mass that is 2 standard deviations below the mean of lean mass for gender specific healthy young adults. In 2010, Cruz-Jentoft AJ et al refined the definition to not only include low muscle mass below 2 standard deviations but either low gait speed (a walking speed below 0.8 meters per second (1.79 miles per hour) in the 4 -minute walk or low muscular strength as measured by grip strength (less than 30 kg in males, less than 20 kg in females). Severe sarcopenia requires the presence of all three conditions (Wikipedia). FYI-normal walking speed is 3.1 miles per hour or 1.4 meters per second.

Falls are the leading cause of fatal and non-fatal injuries for older Americans. One-fourth of Americans aged 65+ fall each year. **One out of five falls cause a serious injury such as broken bones or a** head injury. **One-fourth of seniors who fracture a hip from a fall will die within six months of the injury.** The most profound effect of falling is the loss of independent living. Maintaining adequate muscle mass and avoiding sarcopenia will not solve the problem but may significantly decrease the frequency. Exercise is clearly the best treatment. **Lessening the ravages of muscle mass loss with testosterone may help decrease falling in some people.** Women fall more often than men. The 10-year risk of a cardiovascular event for US men aged 65-69 years is about 28%. We need to compare this to the 10-year risk of falling and fracturing a hip due to poor muscle mass and sarcopenia. The combined lifetime risk for hip, forearm and vertebral fractures coming to clinical attention is around 40%, equivalent to the risk of cardiovascular disease.

The deleterious effects of bed rest on human skeletal muscle fibers are exacerbated by hypercortisolemia and ameliorated by dietary supplementation.

Muscle wasting results from an imbalance between protein synthesis and breakdown. It is generally associated with elevated plasma concentrations of the stress hormone cortisol. A hospitalized patient presents typically in a bedrest environment and a hyper-cortisol endocrine state. Both situations promote protein and muscle breakdown.

This study looked at 28 days of bedrest with three different variables:

1. The first group was simply bedrest.
2. The second group received 5 daily doses of 10-15 mg of oral hydrocortisone to mimic the plasma levels of

cortisol associated with illness or injury (typically cortisol levels of 20 ug/dl).
3. The third group received 16.5 grams of essential amino acids and 30 gm of sucrose dissolved in 250 cc of a noncaloric soft drink (total kcal 558).

The supplemented group maintained body mass and lean leg mass whereas the bedrest group and hyper-cortisol groups lost body mass and muscle mass.

We must always be cognizant of the catabolic environment that a hospitalized patient lives in and encourage protein supplementation and early mobilization (Fitts, et al., 2007).

Testosterone levels and quality of life in diverse male patients with cancers unrelated to androgens.

Symptoms secondary to hormonal changes significantly impact quality of life (QoL) in patients with cancer. This cross-sectional study examines prevalence of hypogonadism and its correlation with QoL and sexual dysfunction.

428 male patients with non-testosterone-related cancer at three cancer centers. Serum was analyzed for total testosterone (TT), free testosterone (FT), bioavailable testosterone (BAT), and sex hormone binding globulin (SHBG). The Functional Assessment of Cancer Therapy-Prostate (FACT-P) QoL questionnaire measured physical, social, emotional, and functional domains as well as sexual function.

Mean and median TTs were 337.46 and 310 ng/dl, respectively. The mean age of patients was 62.05 years.

The crude prevalence of hypogonadism (i.e. TT < 300 ng/dl) was 48%, and mean TT in hypogonadal patients was 176 ng/dl. The prevalences were based on FT (i.e. hypogonadal < 52 pg/dl) and BAT (i.e. hypogonadal < 95 ng/dl) were 78% and 66%, respectively. The mean FT and BAT values in hypogonadal patients were 25 pg/dl and 45 ng/dl, respectively. Hypogonadal patients had decreased total QoL scores on FACT-P ($P = .01$) and decreased three-item sexual function subset.

CONCLUSION:

The prevalence of hypogonadism was unexpectedly high. Measurement of FT or BAT detected a higher prevalence than TT alone, which confirmed previous studies. Correlation of T with FACT-P showed significant reduction of both overall QoL and sexual function for hypogonadal men. BAT and FT levels showed a stronger correlation than TT with overall FACT-P and subscales. **The prevalence of symptomatic hypogonadism in male patients with cancer exceeds that found in comparable studies in noncancer populations** (Fleishman, et al., 2010).

The Association Among Hypogonadism, Symptom Burden, and Survival in Male Patients with Advanced Cancer.

A high frequency of hypogonadism has been reported in male patients with advanced cancer. The current study was performed to evaluate the association between low testosterone levels, symptom burden, and survival in male patients with cancer.

Of 131 consecutive male patients with cancer, 119 (91%) had an endocrine evaluation of total (TT), free (FT), and bioavailable testosterone (BT); high-sensitivity C-reactive protein (CRP); vitamin B12; thyroid-stimulating hormone; 25-hydroxy vitamin D; and cortisol levels when presenting with symptoms of fatigue and/or anorexia-cachexia. The authors examined the correlation using the Spearman test and survival with the log-rank test and Cox regression analysis.

The median age of the patients was 64 years; the majority of patients were white (85 patients; 71%). The median TT level was 209 ng/dL (normal: ≥200 ng/dL), the median FT was 4.4 ng/dL (normal: ≥9 ng/dL), and the median BT was 22.0 ng/dL (normal: ≥61 ng/dL). Low TT, FT, and BT values were all associated with worse fatigue (P≤.04), poor Eastern Cooperative Oncology Group performance status (P≤.05), weight loss (P≤.01), and opioid use (P≤.005). Low TT and FT were associated with increased anxiety (P≤.04), a decreased feeling of well-being (P≤.04), and increased dyspnea (P≤.05), whereas low BT was only found to be associated with anorexia (P=.05). Decreased TT, FT, and BT values were all found to be significantly associated with elevated CRP and low albumin and hemoglobin. On multivariate analysis, decreased survival was associated with low TT (hazards ratio [HR], 1.66; P=.034), declining Eastern Cooperative Oncology Group performance status (HR, 1.55; P=.004), high CRP (HR, 3.28; P<.001), and decreased albumin (HR, 2.52; P<.001).

CONCLUSIONS

In male patients with cancer, low testosterone levels were associated with systemic inflammation, weight loss, increased symptom burden, and decreased survival.

A high frequency of hypogonadism has been reported in male patients with advanced cancer. In the current study, an increased symptom burden, systemic inflammation, weight loss, opioid use, and poor survival were found to be associated with decreased testosterone levels in male patients with cancer. (Dev, et al., 2014).

When and when not to use testosterone for palliation in cancer care.

Hypogonadism is common in patients with cancer. About two thirds of male patients with advanced cancer and more than 70% with cancer cachexia have low testosterone levels compared to 6% of males in the general population (2). Prior to chemotherapy, almost half with metastatic cancer are hypogonadal. 90% of cancer patients taking more than 200 mg morphine or morphine equivalents per day have low T levels. Opioids inhibit FSH, and LH and decrease testicular and adrenal androgen production. The Endocrine Society guidelines recommend measuring testosterone levels in patients requiring long-term opioid therapy (2,4,5,28). Studies have reported increased symptom burden, diminished quality of life, and poor prognosis associated with low testosterone levels in males with cancer. A randomized placebo-controlled trial reported a trend for improved libido, and significantly better performance status after 4 weeks of testosterone treatment (11). Libido seems to improve faster than muscle strength since muscle strength requires several weeks of treatment. Testosterone may relieve symptoms or lessen symptoms of fatigue, hot flashes, poor libido, depression and improve quality of life. By improving performance scores a person may improve his survival chances since many chemotherapies will be adjusted based on low performance scores. The potential benefit seems to far exceed the minimal risk. Although the literature is sparse, and treatment is more controversial, the same idea can help women (Dev, Bruera, & Del Fabbro, 2014).

Effects of Testosterone on Muscle Strength, Physical Function, Body Composition, and Quality of Life in Intermediate-Frail Elderly Men: A Randomized, Double-Blind, Placebo-Controlled Study.

The largest double-blind, placebo-controlled interventional study with T in elderly men to date, the first to investigate its effects in intermediate-frail and frail elderly men. Low T is an important cause of sarcopenia and may therefore contribute to the development of frailty in elderly men. **Frailty is defined by:**

1. unintentional weight loss of 10 lbs. or more in the preceding year.
2. Self-reported exhaustion.
3. Low physical activity.
4. Slow walk time.
5. Low handgrip strength.

274 men at least 65 years old with low or borderline low T levels were randomized to low dose transdermal T (5 mg/d) or placebo gel for 6 months. This improved lower limb muscle strength, increased Lean Body Mass, decreased Fat Mass, and improved somatic and sexual symptoms. T treatment also improved physical function among older (> 75 years) and more frail men.

High-resistance weight training produces greater improvement in muscle strength than pharmacological intervention but usually requires three sessions per week of intense exercise over several months. **T may be a reasonable alternative and is synergistic with exercise** (Srinivas-Shankar, et al., 2010).

Effects of Testosterone on Skeletal Muscle Architecture in Intermediate-Frail and Frail Elderly Men.

30 intermediate-frail and frail elderly men (65-89 years old) with low to borderline-low testosterone levels were enrolled from a single-center randomized, double-blind placebo-controlled trial. Patients received either 50 mg transdermal T gel or placebo gel daily for 6 months. Architecture of the gastrocnemius medialis muscle was assessed by ultrasound imaging at baseline and after 6 months of treatment. **Testosterone treatment resulted in a preservation of muscle thickness at 6 months** while it decreased in the placebo group. **Skeletal muscle retains a high degree of plasticity even into older age** (Atkinson, et al., 2010).

A Randomized Pilot Study of Monthly Cycled Testosterone Replacement or Continuous Testosterone Replacement Versus Placebo in Older Men.

Cycling androgens has been reported by athletes to improve physical performance by enhancing muscle mass and strength. Testosterone traditionally increases skeletal muscle protein synthesis initially but may inhibit skeletal muscle breakdown thus promoting a net anabolism of protein synthesis. This study looked at muscle biopsies looking at muscle protein synthesis and muscle protein breakdown. 24 community-dwelling healthy older men 70 +/- 2 years old with total testosterone levels below 500 ng/dl were randomized into a 5-month double-blind placebo-controlled trial. Subjects were dosed weekly for 5 months, receiving 100 mg testosterone enanthate, or alternating monthly, or placebo.

Total testosterone remained at baseline after each month of placebo and increased after each month of testosterone treatment. Testosterone levels never went out of the normal upper physiological range (1303 ng/dl). Muscle strength for arm curl, arm extension, leg curl, and leg extension increased significantly in the weekly testosterone group. Leg curl strength increased in the monthly group, and there was a trend for strong positive trends in all other muscle groups. There were no changes in one-repetition maximal voluntary strength in the placebo group. Decreased HDL cholesterol occurred in the 2 testosterone groups as noted in other studies of older men. Lean body mass increased in both testosterone groups. The decline in fat mass was significant only in the continuous T group. By raising T levels from the lower half of the normal range in a monthly cycled pattern skeletal muscle synthesis remained consistently elevated in healthy older men. **If monthly on/off cycles of T can consistently increase muscle protein synthesis and lean body mass without an increase in side effects, then this paradigm offers a significant treatment for preventing sarcopenia in older men** (Sheffield-Moore, et al., 2011).

Additive benefit of higher testosterone levels and vitamin D plus calcium supplementation in regard to fall risk reduction among older men and women.

Study investigating the association between sex hormone levels and the risk of falling in older men and women. 199 men and 246 women or older living at home followed for 3 years after baseline assessment of sex hormones.

Men and women in the highest quartile of total testosterone compared to the lowest quartile had a 78% and 66% decreased risk of falling. If individuals also took calcium plus vitamin D the anti-fall effect was enhanced to 84% among men and 85% among women. There was no association of the directly measured free testosterone on falls in both genders (Bischoff-Ferrari, Orav, & Dawson-Hughes, 2008).

Weekly Versus Monthly Testosterone Administration on Fast and Slow Skeletal Muscle Fibers in Older Adult Males.

Loss of mobility due to sarcopenia is exacerbated in men with low T levels.

24 healthy, community-dwelling older men (ages 60-85 years) were randomized into 3 groups for 5 months followed by vastus lateralis muscle(thigh) biopsies. All men had T levels between 204-485 ng/dl. Older men generally have significant muscle atrophy with selective loss of the fast type II muscle fibers, which is considerably more powerful than type I fibers. Type II fibers show the greatest atrophy with age.

The groups were:
1. Eight men receiving weekly 100 mg testosterone ethanate IM.
2. Eight men receiving every other month injections of 100 mg IM weekly
3. Eight men receiving placebo.

This study revealed that monthly T administration increased type II muscle fiber function equally to weekly administration.

T replacement therapy has been shown to protect against losses in muscle mass and strength by increasing muscle protein synthesis and decreasing protein degradation. To prevent large losses in peak power with aging, it is important to reduce atrophy and loss of function in the type II fiber. In that regard, the monthly paradigm is equally as effective as the weekly paradigm with one-half the dose of T (Fitts, et al., 2015).

Lean tissue mass and energy expenditure are retained in hypogonadal men with spinal cord injury after discontinuation of testosterone replacement therapy.

Paralysis after spinal cord injury leads to a dramatic loss of tissue mass (LTM) below the damaged spinal cord level during the first year after acute injury. Disuse atrophy and physical inactivity each contribute to decreased energy expenditure, and without appropriate caloric restriction, result in increased adiposity that may eventually lead to adverse metabolic consequences. Dysfunction of the hypothalamic-pituitary-gonadal axis (HPGA) in persons with spinal code injury may reduce levels of serum testosterone, which may further result in the adverse composition changes. **Low serum T levels are observed in 39-46% of men with spinal cord injury and the percent of low levels are increased for each decade of life compared to the able-bodied male population.** Serum T concentrations have been reported to be inversely related to duration of injury.

Twenty-four healthy non-ambulatory men between the ages of 18 and 65 years old, less than 1 year post-spinal cord injury were enrolled to receive 5-10 mg Testosterone patch (Androderm) for 12 months if their T level was less than 326 mg/dl. 13 subjects received T and 11 were eugonadal. Because of interruption to somatosensory innervation, somatic symptoms of hypogonadism are often not perceived by persons with spinal cord injury.

Individuals were followed 6 months after discontinuation of T therapy with levels decreasing to pre-treatment levels, but what was not anticipated was the retention of lean total mass 6 months after discontinuation of T. The treatment group had significant gains in total body mass (+ 2.7 kg), which persisted 6 months after T treatment. Significant interaction effects were not achieved in the trunk or legs. In the treatment group the trunk increased during treatment. The leg compartment had an increased group mean response during treatment which remained elevated at post-T-treatment compared to the baseline values, but neither of these changes achieved statistical significance. The increase observed in lean total mass (LTM) of the trunk and legs was an unexpected finding because of the presence of muscle paralysis and immobility in the lower extremities and portions of the trunk.

Six months after discontinuation of T treatment beneficial changes persisted to LTM, energy expenditure, and possibly HDL level (Bauman, La Fountaine, Cirnigliaro, Kirshblum, & Spungen, 2015).

Multiple hormonal dysregulation as determinant of low physical performance and mobility in older persons.

Abstract
Mobility-disability is a common condition in older individuals. Many factors, including the age-related hormonal dysregulation, may concur to the development of disability in the elderly. In fact, during the aging process it is observed an imbalance between anabolic hormones that decrease (testosterone, dehydroepiandrosterone sulphate (DHEAS), estradiol, insulin like growth factor-1 (IGF-1) and Vitamin D) and catabolic hormones (cortisol, thyroid hormones) that increase. The studies ranged from 2002 to 2013, and the age of the participants (≥65 years). We hypothesized that the parallel decline of anabolic hormones has a higher impact than a single hormonal derangement on adverse mobility outcomes in older population. Given the multifactorial origin of low mobility, we underlined the need of future synergistic optional treatments (micronutrients and exercise) to improve the effectiveness of hormonal treatment and to safely ameliorate the anabolic hormonal status and mobility in older individuals (Maggio, et al., 2014).

Vitamin D deficiency, muscle function, and falls in elderly people.

Vitamin D has well-known effects on bone metabolism but deficiency is also associated with weakness, predomi-

SARCOPENIA (POVERTY OF THE FLESH)

nately of the proximal muscle groups. Experimental findings have shown;

1. Vitamin D supplementation in vitamin D-deficient, elderly people improved muscle strength, walking distance, and functional ability and resulted in a reduction of falls and nonvertebral fractures.
2. In healthy elderly people, muscle strength declined with age and was not prevented by vitamin D supplementation.
3. Severe comorbidity might affect muscle strength in such a way that restoration of a good vitamin D status has a limited effect on functional ability.
4. An elevated intact PTH level is a common indicator of vitamin D deficiency. Caution should be exercised when an elevated serum PTH is used as an indicator of vitamin D deficiency since physical inactivity increases bone turnover and serum concentrations, which prevents an elevation in serum PTH, even in the presence of vitamin D deficiency. **Both an elevated PTH level and normal PTH can occur with vitamin D deficiency** (Janssen, Samson, & Verhaar, 2002)

Aerobic reserve and physical functional performance in older adults.

29 men and 23 women aged 70-92 years old performed physical tests while measuring peak oxygen consumption. In older adults, performance of daily tasks requires between 30 and 50% of aerobic capacity. Light household

tasks and carrying groceries require moderate (40-60%) aerobic intensity. **Aerobic capacity between 18 and 20 ml/kg/min has been defined as an aerobic threshold below which there is a reduced probability of living independently.** Older adults with little or no aerobic reserve may be perilously close to, or fall below, minimum physiological thresholds required to perform daily tasks. A higher aerobic reserve provides older adults with a larger margin of safety. Having a larger aerobic reserve allows an older person to engage in more leisurely or pleasurable activities/hobbies rather than just surviving. **Testosterone could be that variable that keeps a person's reserve above the dangerous downhill spiral.**

Healthy VO2max levels(ml/kg/min)	Men	Women
Age 50-59 years	39-43	33-37
60-69	36-39	30-33
70-79	32-37	28-30
Unhealthy below 18-20		

(Arnett, Laity, Agrawal, & Cress, 2008)

Age-Related Decline in Maximal Oxygen Capacity: Consequences for Performance of Everyday Activities.

A minimum aerobic threshold for independent living appears to fluctuate between 13 and 15 ml 02/min/kg, which has been suggested as a minimum requirement for successfully coping with everyday tasks. Nine young women (32.2 years old), eight middle-aged (54.1 years), and eight old (77 years) Danish women were studied. Elderly women experience O2 consumption during everyday activities near their VO2max, whereas middle-aged and young subjects possess a more significant margin between these two parameters. VO2max is reported to decrease 5% to 15% after age 25. The present study revealed an even more significant decrease of 29% between the young and the middle-aged groups (14.5% decline per decade) and 27% between the middle-aged and the old groups (10.8% decline per decade).

Oxygen consumption during performance of everyday activities was similar in the different age groups of women. In contrast, a significant age-related decline in VO2max was noticed. **Our oxygen capacity and reserve decrease dramatically as we age eventually making everyday tasks such as stair climbing, walking, dressing, and vacuuming difficult and finally impossible to perform.** Getting old is just not fun! Exercise, exercise, exercise (Puggaard, 2005).

Protein Ingestion Prior to Strength Exercise Affects Blood Hormones and Metabolism.

Ten resistance-trained young men consumed either a 25-gram whey/caseinate protein or a noncaloric placebo 30 minutes before a heavy strength training session (STS) in a crossover design separated by at least 7 days. A protein-carbohydrate supplement was consumed after STS in both trials. Blood samples for growth hormone, testosterone, and free fatty acids were drawn before, during and after STS. Consuming 25 grams of whey/caseinate protein 30 minutes before an STS significantly decreased serum

Growth hormone, testosterone and free fatty acid levels, and increased serum insulin during an STS. The pre-STS protein increased EPOC (excess post-exercise oxygen consumption) and RER (respiratory exchange ratio) significantly during two-hour recovery after STS. RER compares the CO2 produced with metabolism with the oxygen consumed.

Basic science information-Amino acid availability is important for muscle protein synthesis. Hyper-aminoacidemia with an increase in insulin at a time when blood flow is increased appears to offer the maximum stimulation of muscle protein synthesis. Protein supplementation (mostly whey) before and after an STS is advantageous for gaining muscle size compared with carbohydrates. Whey and casein/caseinate are popular proteins among strength athletes, and both have recently been shown to be effective in increasing net muscle protein balance after an STS.

Enhanced insulin levels resulting from the protein ingestion before exercise could be expected to have a favorable effect on net protein balance because insulin is generally accepted as a stimulator of protein synthesis only when adequate amino acids are available. This was presumably the case in the Protein trial because of the consumed protein drink before the STS increased the blood insulin during the STS to levels that have been suggested to maximally stimulate muscle protein synthesis. Whey and caseins both significantly increase blood amino acid levels. Resistance exercise has been shown to result in acute elevations of T that peak early after exercise and return to baseline by about 60-minutes post-exercise.

In conclusion, the study indicated that consuming 25 grams of whey/caseinate protein 30 minutes before heavy STS will provide the muscle a more anabolic environment by increasing the serum insulin levels during an STS and possibly by increased testosterone uptake into the muscle (Hulmi, Volek, Selänne, & Mero, 2005).

Hormonal Responses and Adaptations to Resistance Exercise and Training.

With progressive overload, muscle motor unit recruitment will increase. Recruitment of a greater number of muscle fibers enables greater hormone-tissue interaction within the realm of a larger percentage of the total muscle mass. **Tissue remodeling is a dual process in that catabolism initiates the process during resistance exercise and anabolism predominates in the recovery period leading to growth and repair.** Resistance exercise has been shown to acutely increase total testosterone concentrations in most studies in men, while in young women no change or an elevation may take place. Free testosterone has been shown to be elevated by 25% in young women following acute resistance exercise; however, no changes have been observed following resistance exercise in middle-aged and elderly women. It appears that programs designed to stimulate testosterone secretion should be structured around large muscle-mass exercises. **Men have shown acute elevations in testosterone but not women immediately following the same protocol. It appears other anabolic hormones such as GH may be more influential for promoting muscle hypertrophy in women.**

Long-term studies have shown no further improvement in muscle strength or hypertrophy with DHEA/androstenedione/androstenediol supplementation (150-300 md/day) over 8-12 weeks of resistance training. The subsequent elevations in testosterone metabolites, estradiol, estrone, and reductions in HDLs potentially pose health risks that need to be considered prior to prohormone use.

Resistance exercise has been shown to elevate the concentrations of human GH through 30-minutes post-exercise similarly in men and women, although the resting concentrations of GH are significantly higher in women.

Glucocorticoids are released from the adrenal cortex in response to the stress of exercise. Cortisol has catabolic functions that have greater effects in type II muscle fibers. In peripheral tissues, cortisol stimulates lipolysis in adipose cells and increases protein degradation and decreases protein synthesis in muscle cells resulting in greater release of lipids and amino acids into circulation. While chronic high levels of cortisol have adverse effects, acute elevations may be part of a larger remodeling process in muscle tissue. Ingestion of carbohydrates, amino acids, or combinations of both prior to, during, and or immediately after the resistance exercise protocol is recommended for maximizing insulin's effect on tissue anabolism. **Supplementation prior to or during resistance exercise is especially beneficial for maximizing protein synthesis because it takes advantage of the large increase in muscular blood flow and subsequent amino acid delivery.** Men who are considered obese have been shown to have low concentrations of total and free testosterone, SHBG and SHBG binding capacity with the magnitude directly related to the level of body fat. Leptin concentrations are highly correlated to body fat mass such that obese humans have on average four times more serum leptin than lean individuals (Kraemer & Ratamess, 2005).

Aging of endocrine system and its potential impact on sarcopenia.

After the age of 35 years, a physiological decline of muscle mass occurs at an annual rate of 1-2% with a 1.5% per year reduction in strength, which accelerates around 3% after the age of 60 years.

1. **Estrogens** are very important for bone density both in men and women. One has to look at cost-benefit ratio between protecting bone density versus increasing risk of breast cancer and stroke. The lowest possible estrogen dose to alleviate symptoms is the general rule.
2. **DHEA (Dehydroepiandrosterone)** is a natural steroid and precursor hormone produced by the adrenal glands and transformed to androgens or estrogens in several tissues. **A recent systematic review based on eight randomized controlled trials selected from 155 eligible studies, reported that no benefit of oral DHEA supplementation on muscle strength and physical function in older subjects was consistently found.**
3. **Vitamin D**. Vitamin D supplementation is simple enough and probably mostly beneficial. Because it is

fat-soluble, it can accumulate if very high doses are routinely given without levels checked. Many times, nursing home residents will have single digit levels and 50,000 units several times per week is prescribed. The important concept is to check levels when high doses are given. A systematic meta-analysis performed on 30 randomized controlled trials showed that vitamin D supplementation induced a small but significant increase in muscle strength, particularly on the lower limb, but with no improvement in muscle mass However, the effects of vitamin D on the risk of falls are still a matter of debate due to contradictory results. In 2011, a meta-analysis reported that vitamin D alone had no effect on falls, whereas vitamin D combined with calcium reduced the odds of falling by 17% compared with placebo/controls. A 2014 meta-analysis showed that vitamin D supplementation, with or without calcium, does not reduce the incidence of falls by more than 15%.

4. **Growth hormone (GH), Insulin-like growth factor-1 (IGF-1).** Daily GH production has been reported to decline by 14% per decade after the age of 30 years, with a parallel decline in IGF-1 secretion. (Vitale, Cesari, & Mari, 2016)

Off-label use of hormones as an antiaging strategy: a review

Despite evident positive effects in adolescents and adults with GH-deficiency, long-term GH therapy to prevent and treat sarcopenia in elderly individuals with low GH/IGF-1 levels related to age is still unclear. (Samaras, Papadopoulou, Samaras, & Ongaro, 2014)

Melatonin as a Potential Agent in the Treatment of Sarcopenia

Worldwide estimates predict 2 billion people will be over 65 years old by 2050. Of all the degenerative processes, the development of limitations in mobility is one of the most common, leading to a reduced capacity for daily living activities, disability and loss of independence. Sarcopenia, however, not only refers to muscle mass deterioration; numerous other factors are involved in the reduction in muscle quality associated with aging. These include derangement of skeletal myocytes, vascular dysfunction, reduced aerobic capacity, fat infiltration and a decline in bone mineral density.

Melatonin, is a derivative of tryptophan, an essential amino acid. It is produced by the pineal gland in a circadian manner with maximal production during the night. This molecule has important protective capabilities, mainly based on its high potency as a free radical scavenger.

- Pineal production and plasma melatonin levels progressively drop during aging to the extent that in advanced age its levels are almost null.
- The rise in oxidative stress in sarcopenia is mainly a result of mitochondrial dysfunction.
- Melatonin, in its role as a homeostasis stabilizer, has been shown to induce or reduce autophagy in muscles of sarcopenic patients
- Melatonin reduces endoplasmic reticulum stress in skeletal muscle by increasing the expression of several proteins as well as mRNA levels; this improves protein

synthesis. Likewise, melatonin is an important regulator of proteasome and lysosomal mechanisms, thereby enhancing cell quality.
- The anti-inflammatory actions of melatonin are well-documented in numerous organs.
- With regard to supplementation with melatonin, firstly, no significant adverse effects have been reported with its use at any concentration or at any treatment time
- In contrast, a long-term treatment with melatonin has vasculoprotective properties

Bone and muscle are closely interrelated. Thus, when aging affects one of these two tissues, the functionality of the other is likewise compromised. Thus, as muscle quality deteriorates during aging, also bone becomes weakened when it develops osteoporosis.

The reliance of muscle health on bone and vice versa is so interrelated that several researchers consider it one syndrome, with terms including sarco-osteopenia, sarco-osteoporosis, or dysmobility syndrome to distinguish disorders which are prone to a high risk of fractures.

While still limited, the scientific evidence is consistent in terms of suggesting that melatonin significantly improves aged muscle as well as other cellular alterations characteristic of sarcopenia.

Conclusions

Sarcopenia is a highly burdensome geriatric syndrome. It is commonly associated with osteoporosis and neuromuscular dysfunction. Currently, no effective treatment for this degenerative process has been identified. Melatonin has a high safety profile and no serious toxicity related to melatonin usage has been reported. Here, we summarized the scientific evidence that melatonin prevents and counteracts mitochondrial impairments, reduces oxidative stress and autophagic alterations in muscle cells, increases the number of satellite cells and limits sarcopenic changes in skeletal muscle. Likewise, melatonin lowers chronic low inflammation levels and reduces vascular aging, all of which are usually present in sarcopenic muscle. Similarly, melatonin improves the endocrine signaling which deteriorates in aged individuals. **Much of the research involved animal model systems**. (Coto-Montes, Boga, Tan, & Reiter, 2016)

Exercise

WHAT CAN I SAY ABOUT exercise? The benefits of exercise are profound and everyone agrees. Exercise is a key component of general health, weight loss and maintenance of weight loss. People who succeed at maintaining a healthy weight make exercise a large part of their life. Unfortunately, many people do not like exercising. Exercise is usually defined as planned or structured physical activity and involves repetitive bodily movements. It has a start and a finish. People do not have to formally exercise but need to increase their physical activity. Physical activity simply means any movement which burns calories. One does not need to exercise 40 minutes continuously, but many can do physical activity 10 minutes at a time, 4 times per day. Developing lifelong positive behaviors promotes success. Physical activity and exercise may generate a net effect on energy balance much greater than the direct energy cost of the activity alone. Many studies of human subjects indicate beneficial effects lasting up to 48 hours

If exercise is so great, then why do so few people partake? The answer is easy- it is hard. When was the last time you say a runner on the street smiling? What is more fun having a bowl of ice cream or breathing hard and sweating? I have some patients tell me that they do not mind exercising if they don't have to sweat. If someone is not brought up exercising, then exercising is like learning a foreign language.

EXERCISE

    I exercise for many reasons. One reason is to prepare myself to handle an illness both physically and mentally when it happens. One day I will be weak and frail. How a person responds to an illness or surgery speaks volumes about their health. For instance, if one gets released from the hospital in 2 days from a knee replacement versus going to a skilled nursing facility for 2 weeks. Many patients do not have insight about how difficult major or minor surgery can be. Sometimes, I wish I could say that surgery is like a man or woman coming at you with a very sharp knife while you are asleep and the person is very good with the knife too. Of course, this is just a silly analogy but it still amazes me how unrealistic some people are. I also exercise to maintain muscle mass. Exercise releases endogenous endorphins that make people feel good and is a very strong stimulus for growth hormone which gives me the irrational idea that I will live forever. One of the problems with getting older is the idea of feeling invincible goes away. As you get older you lose that feeling. It sometimes returns after a good workout but becomes less and less often. When I exercise I see an old man that no longer flows like liquid but looks and feels like a stick figure. Instead of being smooth and flowing like a ballet dancer, I am more like a stiff-legged person. I'm just buying time till my next nuisance injury that makes me slower than I already feel. The idea that I am in better shape than 98% of people my age provides no comfort at all. I get discouraged at times but always remember to never quit. It is like the old Woody Allen phrase "I feel life is divided into the horrible and the miserable. That's the two categories. The horrible are like, terminal cases, you know, blind people, crippled. I don't know how they get through life. It's amazing to me. And the miserable is everyone else. So, you should be thankful that you're miserable, because that's very lucky, to be miserable."

Dr. James Gibney wrote an article how fuel works in our bodies. It is beautifully written and flows very well. That is not a description of my body anymore. Embrace the paragraph.

The ability to perform exercise requires combustion of metabolic fuels, transforming chemical into kinetic and thermal energy. Glucose is the preferred fuel source for short-term high-intensity activity, whereas FFAs (derived from the circulation or from TG stored in muscle or adipose tissue) become increasingly important during more prolonged activity. O2 delivery to muscles depends upon adequate ventilation and O2 transport to hemoglobin, circulatory distribution by an adequate cardiac output and peripheral circulation, dilatation of the muscle capillary network, and extraction of O2 by the muscle fibers with either storage in myoglobin or immediate combustion. GH could improve exercise performance through increased delivery of substrate and oxygen to exercising muscle, increased muscle strength, or a combination of these variables. GH could also improve exercise performance through indirect mechanisms, including changes in body composition or more efficient thermoregulation. (Gibney, Healy, & Sönksen, 2007)

Resistance training with weights will not promote clinically significant weight loss but is very helpful for ADLs (activities of daily living) and helps maintain muscle mass. Resistance training has been shown to increase HDL by 8-21%, decrease LDL by 13-23% and reduce TG by 11-18%. Statistics show 25% of individuals do no physical activity and 50% do insufficient physical activity. A simple test to assess the intensity of exercise is the "talk test." Low intensity allows one to talk comfortably or sing. Moderate intensity allows fragmented talk and high intensity exercise the person is not able to speak. People that exercise want to procrastinate or make excuses like everyone else but they don't because they deeply believe the benefits outweigh the hassle.

A 2012 article entitled **Exercise acts as a drug; the pharmacological benefits of exercise** by J Vina in the British Journal of Pharmacology expresses some insight.

> The beneficial effects of regular exercise for the promotion of health and cure of diseases have been clearly shown. **Exercise is so effective that it should be considered as a drug. As with any drug, dosing is very important**. More attention needs be paid to the dosing and to individual variations between patients. **The philosopher Plato (427-347BC) said "Lack of activity destroys the good condition of every human being while movement and methodical physical exercise saves and preserves it."** (Myers, et al., 2004; Vina, Sanchis-Gomar, Martinez-Bello, & Gomez-Cabrera, 2012)
>
> Modest increments in energy expenditure due to physical activity (about 1000 kcal per week) or an increase in physical fitness of 1 MET (metabolic equivalent) is associated with lowering mortality by about 20% (Myers, et al., 2004).
>
> Both resistance and aerobic training have been shown to be of benefit for the control of diabetes; however, resistance training may have greater benefits for glycemic control than aerobic training (Dunstan, et al., 2005).

Wen, et al., **2011** noted that 15 minutes a day or 90 minutes a week of moderate-intensity exercise is of benefit in terms of life expectancy, even for subjects with cardiovascular risks. Moderate-intensity activities are those in which heart rate and breathing are raised; but, still, it is possible to speak comfortably. This occurs around 4-6 METS and brisk walking at 3 mph is one such activity.

A dose-response relation appears to exist, such that people who have the highest levels of physical activity and fitness are at lowest risk of premature death (Warburton, Nicol, & Bredin, 2006). Having said that, less active men who participate in vigorous activity were more likely to have a myocardial infarction during exercise than the most active men (Thompson, et al., 2007). "You don't run before you walk."

In the pharmacological treatment of many conditions, physicians typically start with a dose of a drug believed to be the minimum effective dose. The intensity of aerobic training may be also titrated in healthy people. As with medicines, special considerations should be taken when prescribing exercise for people with special needs such as elderly, children, pregnant women, overweight or obese patients and patients with chronic diseases.

Exercise causes a significant reduction in cancer rates, specifically colon and breast cancer (Shephard & Futcher, 1997) (Pederson, 2006).

Exercise acts as an antioxidant, because training increases the expression of antioxidant enzymes (Gomez-Cabrera, Domenech, & Viña, 2008).

An interesting study in the International Journal Sports Medicine looked at high intensity exercise in 2011. It is widely held among the general population and even among medical professionals that moderate exercise is a healthy practice but long term high intensity exercise is not. The specific amount of physical activity necessary for good health remains unclear. F. Sanchis-Gomar and others studied the longevity of 834 Tour de France cyclists from France (465), Belgium (173), and Italy (196), between 1930 and 1964 with death rates up till December 31, 2007 compared with the pooled general population of France, Belgium, and Italy for comparative ages. A very significant increase in average longevity (17%) of the cyclists were noted compared to the general population. **The age at which 50% of the general population died was 73.5 years compared to 81.5 years in Tour de France participants.** (Sanchis-Gomar, Olaso-Gonzalez, Corella, Gomez-Cabrera, & Vina, 2011)

Another study, entitled **<u>Lifelong Physical Activity Regardless of Dose Is Not Associated with Myocardial Fibrosis</u>**, refuted the suggestion that long-term intensive physical training may be associated with adverse cardiovascular effects, including the development of myocardial fibrosis.

> 92 seniors (mean age 69 years, 27% women) free of major chronic illnesses who engaged in stable physical activity over 25 years were classified into 4 groups by the number of sessions/week of aerobic activity.
>
> Group 1 less than two 30 minute sessions per week.
> Group 2 2-3 sessions/week.
> Group 3 4-5 sessions/week.
> Group 4 6-7 sessions/week.

All subjects underwent cardiopulmonary exercise testing and cardiac magnetic resonance imaging, including late gadolinium enhancement assessment of fibrosis. Cardiac imaging demonstrated increasing left ventricular end-diastolic volumes, end systolic volumes, stroke volumes, with increasing doses of lifelong physical activity.

A lifelong history of consistent physical activity, regardless of dose ranging from sedentary to competitive marathon running, was not associated with the development of focal myocardial fibrosis. (Abdullah, et al., 2016)

A prospective cohort study looking at all-cause mortality in 204,542 Australian adults aged 45 through 75 years old over an 8-year period looking at death rate and amount of moderate to vigorous exercise activity was published in JAMA 2015.

1. Low time 10-149 minutes/week. Death rate 4.81%
2. Moderate time 150-299 minutes/week. Death rate 3.17%
3. Large time 300 minutes/week or more. Death rate 2.64%

There was an inverse dose-response relationship between proportion of vigorous activity and mortality. (Gebel, et al., 2015)

Few strategies have been effective in treating the rapid rise in obesity worldwide. A study presently being conducted by will focus on preventing excessive weight gain rather than weight reduction: **Evaluating a small change approach to preventing long term weight gain in overweight and obese adults.**

> Individuals will reduce overall energy balance by 100-200 kcal per day by reducing calorie intake and/or increase daily step count by 2000 per day (2000 steps is about 100 kcals). The primary outcome is change in body weight and body composition. 320 primarily white (305) overweight and obese men and women are randomized to Usual care or Small change approach. The intervention is two years with a one year follow-up. (Ross, Hill, Latimer, & Day, 2016)
>
> In some people, the reality may be to prevent more weight gain rather than weight loss. Although not as glamorous as weight loss, this could be very helpful for millions.

Physical exercise as a preventive or disease-modifying treatment of dementia and brain aging

> A rapidly growing literature strongly suggests that exercise, specifically aerobic exercise, may attenuate cognitive impairment and reduce dementia risk. The idea of neuroplasticity is an evolving concept that has important implications in disease prevention and treatment. Meta-analysis and randomized controlled trials have shown the following:
>
> 1. significantly reduced risk of dementia associated with midlife exercise.
> 2. midlife exercise significantly reduced later risks of mild cognitive impairment.

3. among patients with dementia or mild cognitive impairment 6-12 months of exercise documented better cognitive scores compared with sedentary controls.
4. aerobic exercise in healthy adults were associated with significantly improved cognitive scores.
5. one year of aerobic exercise in seniors was associated with significantly larger hippocampal volumes and better spatial memory.
6. physically fit seniors had significantly larger hippocampal or gray matter volumes compared with unfit seniors.
7. brain cognitive networks studied using functional magnetic resonance imaging display improved connectivity after 6 to 12 months of exercise.
8. animal studies indicate that exercise facilitates neuroplasticity via a variety of biomechanisms, with improved learning outcomes.

Besides a brain neuroprotective effect, physical exercise may also attenuate cognitive decline via mitigation of cerebrovascular risk, including the contribution of small vessel disease to dementia. Exercise should not be overlooked as an important therapeutic strategy. (Ahlskog, Geda, Graff-Radford, & Petersen, 2011)

Aerobic Fitness in late adolescence and the risk of early death

In the International Journal of Epidemiology researchers followed 1.3 million Swedish men from time of mandatory conscription (age 18) in 1969-1996 through 2012. Aerobic fitness was assessed with a cycle test. During roughly 29 years of follow-up, over 44,000 men died. Men in the highest fifth of aerobic fitness at baseline had a 41% lower risk for all-cause mortality than those in the lowest fifth. **The benefits of fitness decreased with increasing baseline BMI, with no protective effect seen at BMIs of 35 or greater.** In addition, mortality risk was 30% lower among unfit normal-weight men than fit obese men (Högström, Nordström, & Nordström, 2016).

This provides evidence against "fat but fit." **Being obese but "physically fit" helps but does not protect you from the increase in mortality compared to non-obese people.**

Exercise Training and Nutritional Supplementation for Physical Frailty in Very Elderly People.

Randomized, placebo-controlled trial comparing progressive resistance exercise training, multi-nutrient supplementation, both interventions and neither interventions in 100 frail nursing home residents with an average age of 87 years old (range 72 to 98) over a 10-week period. Muscle strength increased 113%, gait velocity increased by 11.8%, stair-climbing power by 28.4% compared to less than 5% increase or decline in non-exercisers. In contrast, **multi-nutrient supplementation without concomitant exercise does not reduce muscle weakness or physical frailty**. Several studies have shown acquisition of maximal strength, even in patients of advanced age and those with chronic disease the superiority of high-intensity, dynamic resistance training for them. **The aging musculoskeletal system retains its responsiveness to progressive resis-**

tance training, and most important, the correction of disuse is accompanied by significant improvement in the levels of functional mobility and overall activity (Fiatarone, et al., 1994).

Minimum amount of physical activity for reduced mortality and extended life expectancy: a prospective cohort study.

Prospective cohort study of 416,175 individuals (199,265 men and 216,910 women) were followed an average of 8.05 years with a self-administered questionnaire dividing participants into five categories of exercise. **Those in the low volume group consisting of 15 minutes per day had a 14% reduced risk of all-cause mortality and had a 3 year longer life expectancy compared to the sedentary group. Any amount of exercise is better than none** (Wen, et al., 2011).

Light Intensity Physical Activity and Sedentary Behavior in Relation to Body Mass Index and Grip Strength in Older Adults: Cross-Sectional Findings from the Lifestyle Interventions and Independence for Elders (Life) Study.

Hypothesis- light intensity activities, such as walking or light housework, contribute to energy expenditure and may therefore contribute to lowering fat mass levels by improving energy balance to energy expenditure.

1,635 participants with 67% women aged 70-89 years old with heightened risk of mobility/disability yet able to walk 400 meters in 15 minutes without sitting, leaning or assistance from a walker or another person wore an accelerometer for seven consecutive days to assess energy expenditure. **The study showed that greater time spent** in light intensity activity and lower sedentary times (for example watching TV) were associated with lower BMI (Bann, et al., 2013).

Strategic creatine supplementation and resistance training in healthy older adults.

Sarcopenia, the age-related loss of muscle mass and strength decreases the ability to perform activities of daily living. Creatine supplementation was compared to placebo in a double-blind study in older adults (50-71 years old). (Creatine is a nitrogen source that promotes ATP formation which provides energy for reactions). A typical person makes 1 gram per day which comes from our diet.

64 older adults (38 postmenopausal women, 26 men) were randomized to receive creatine (0.1 gm/kg) immediately before exercise followed by placebo after exercise, or placebo both before and after exercise, or placebo followed by creatine after exercise for 32 weeks. A creatine dose of 0.1 gm/kg was chosen because it increases muscle mass and strength without causing adverse effects in young and older adults. Of the 64 participants enrolled, 39 completed the study (22 females, 17 males).

This is the first study to directly compare creatine supplementation before and after resistance training with a placebo in healthy older adults.

Results showed that:
1. Creatine supplementation increased muscle strength over placebo.
2. Post-exercise creatine increased lean tissue mass more than placebo and pre-exercise creatine.

3. Creatine increased upper and lower body strength compared with resistance training alone.

(Candow, Vogt, Johannsmeyer, Forbes, & Farthing, 2015)

Suppression of endogenous testosterone production attenuates the response to strength training: a randomized, placebo-controlled, and blinded intervention study.

Abstract

We hypothesized that suppression of endogenous testosterone (GnRH which suppresses T) would inhibit the adaptations to strength training in otherwise healthy men. Twenty-two young men with minor experience with strength training participated in this randomized, placebo-controlled, double-blinded intervention study. The subjects were randomized to treatment with the GnRH analog goserelin (3.6 mg) or placebo (saline) subcutaneously every 4 wk for 12 wk. The strength training period of 8 wk, starting at week 4, included exercises for all major muscles [3-4 sets per exercise x 6-10 repetitions with corresponding 6- to 10-repetition maximum (RM) loads, 3/wk].

Endogenous testosterone decreased significantly ($P < 0.01$) in the goserelin group from 22.6 nmol/l to 2.0 (week 4) and 1.1 nmol/l (week 12), whereas it remained constant in the placebo group. The goserelin group showed no changes in isometric knee extension strength after training, whereas the placebo group increased from 240.2 to 264.1 Nm ($P < 0.05$ within and $P = 0.05$ between groups). Lean mass of the legs increased 0.37 and 0.57

kg in the goserelin and placebo groups, respectively (P < 0.05 within and P = 0.05 between groups). Body fat mass increased 1.4 kg and decreased 0.6 kg in the goserelin and placebo groups, respectively (P < 0.05 within and between groups). **We conclude that endogenous testosterone is of paramount importance to the adaptation to strength training. It's hard enough to work-out after a long day but then to know that one's effort has diminished return is discouraging** (Kvorning, Andersen, Brixen, & Madsen, 2006).

2014 National statistics for U.S. community hospital stays.

Knee arthroplasty	723,086
Total and partial hip arthroplasty	505,170
Spinal fusion	414,611
Treatment fracture or dislocation of hip and femur	257,36

(Healthcare Cost and Utilization Project (HCUP), 2014)

International Osteoporosis Foundation

- A 10% loss of bone mass in the vertebrae can double the risk of vertebral fractures, and similarly, a 10% loss of bone mass in the hip can result in a 2.5 times greater risk of hip fracture.
- Worldwide, 1 in 3 women over age 50 will experience osteoporotic fractures, as will 1 in 5 men aged over 50.
- The combined lifetime risk for hip, forearm, and vertebral fractures coming to clinical attention is around 40%, equivalent to the risk for cardiovascular disease.

- Although the overall prevalence of fragility fractures is higher in women, men generally have higher rates of fracture related mortality.
- In women over 45 years of age, osteoporosis accounts for more days spent in the hospital than many other diseases, including diabetes, myocardial infarction, and breast cancer.

Hip fractures cause the most morbidity with reported mortality rates up to 20-24% in the first year after a hip fracture, and greater risk of dying may persist for at least 5 years afterwards. Loss of function and independence among survivors is profound, with 40% unable to walk independently, 60% requiring assistance a year later. Because of these losses, 33% are totally dependent or in a nursing home in the year following a hip fracture. Up to 20% of patients die in the first year following hip fractures, mostly due to pre-existing medical conditions. **Less than half those who survive the hip fracture regain their previous level of function.**

Proton pump inhibiting drugs can reduce the absorption of calcium from the stomach and long-term use of these drugs can significantly increase the risk of an osteoporosis-related fracture.

Supplementation with vitamin D has improved lower extremity muscle performance and reduced risk of falling in several high-quality double blind randomized control trials.

Osteoporosis and low bone mass are currently estimated to be a major public health threat for almost 44 million U.S. women and men aged 50 and older. This represents 55% of people aged 50 and older in the United States. (International Osteoporosis Foundation, 2017)

Interventions to Slow Aging in Humans: Are We Ready?

A consensus of experts agreed on the following points

1. Aging can be slowed by many interventions.
2. Slowing aging typically delays or prevents a range of chronic diseases of old age.
3. Dietary, nutraceuticals and pharmacologic interventions that modulate relevant intracellular signaling pathways and can be considered for human intervention have been identified. Additional potential targets will continue to emerge as research progresses.
4. It is now necessary to cautiously proceed to test these interventions in humans.

The strategies believed to be the most promising are

1. Pharmacological inhibition of the GH/IGF-1 axis.
2. Protein restriction and fasting diets.
3. Pharmacological inhibition of the TOR-S6K pathway (involved in cell growth and proliferation.)
4. Pharmacological regulation of certain sirtuin proteins (proteins speculated to promote longevity) and the use of spermidine (possible longevity agent) and other epigenetic modulators.
5. Pharmacological inhibition of inflammation.
6. Chronic metformin use.

I thought choices 2,5, and 6 were interesting. Although the effects of chronic cycles of prolonged fasting on life span is not known, these studies point to prolonged fasting, which could be carried out in humans as infrequently as once a month of less, as a potent inducer of protective systems and a potential alternative to chronic calorie reduction and intermittent or alternate day fasting. **Part of the protective effects of fasting against aging and disease may be mediated by the reduction in IGF-1, glucose, and insulin** (Longo, et al., 2015).

Dysfunctional endogenous analgesia during exercise in patients with chronic pain: to exercise or not to exercise?

Abstract
BACKGROUND:
Exercise is an effective treatment for various chronic pain disorders, including fibromyalgia, chronic neck pain, osteoarthritis, rheumatoid arthritis, and chronic low back pain. Although the clinical benefits of exercise therapy in these populations are well established (i.e. evidence based), it is currently unclear whether exercise has positive effects on the processes involved in chronic pain (e.g. central pain modulation).
OBJECTIVES:
Reviewing the available evidence addressing the effects of exercise on central pain modulation in patients with chronic pain.
METHODS:
Narrative review.

RESULTS:

Exercise activates endogenous analgesia in healthy individuals. The increased pain threshold following exercise is due to the release of endogenous opioids and activation of (supra)spinal nociceptive inhibitory mechanisms orchestrated by the brain. Exercise triggers the release of beta-endorphins from the pituitary (peripherally) and the hypothalamus (centrally), which in turn enables analgesic effects by activating μ-opioid receptors peripherally and centrally, respectively. The hypothalamus, has the capacity to activate descending nociceptive inhibitory mechanisms. However, several groups have shown dysfunctioning of endogenous analgesia in response to exercise in patients with chronic pain. Muscle contractions activate generalized endogenous analgesia in healthy, pain-free humans and patients with either osteoarthritis or rheumatoid arthritis, but result in increased generalized pain sensitivity in fibromyalgia patients. In patients having local muscular pain (e.g. shoulder myalgia), exercising non-painful muscles activates generalized endogenous analgesia. However, exercising painful muscles does not change pain sensitivity either in the exercising muscle or at distant locations.

LIMITATIONS:

The reviewed studies examined acute effects of exercise rather than long-term effects of exercise therapy.

CONCLUSIONS:

A dysfunctional response of patients with chronic pain and aberrations in central pain modulation to exercise has been shown, indicating that exercise therapy should be individually tailored with emphasis on prevention of symptom flares (Nijs, Kosek, Van Oosterwijck, & Meeus, 2012).

Inflammation and the gut

CHRONIC, LOW-GRADE INFLAMMATION IS RECOGNIZED as a major characteristic of aging. This phenomenon is so pervasive that the term "inflammaging" has been coined to emphasize that many major age-related disabilities, including cancers, susceptibility to infections, and dementia have immunopathogenic components. "Inflammaging" appears to be much more complex than previously thought, and a variety of tissues and organs participate in producing inflammatory stimuli. The list is extensive and includes the immune system, but also adipose tissue, skeletal muscle, liver, and the gut. The gut is of unique importance, because it is the body's largest immune organ and contains trillions of bacteria that can release inflammatory stimuli into the portal and systemic circulation.

Two reviews provide summaries;

The contributory role of gut microbiota in cardiovascular disease.

The human gut harbors more than 100 trillion microbial cells, far outnumbering the human host cells of the body. We are the minority shareholders in our body. Homo sapiens DNA is estimated to represent less than 10% of the total DNA within our bodies, due to the staggeringly large numbers of microbes that reside in and on us, primarily within our gut. The major taxa present in gut microbiota consist primarily of 2 major bacterial phyla, Firmicutes and Bacteroidetes, whose proportions appear to remain remarkably stable over time within individuals and their family members. However, the composition of the remaining gut microbiota is remarkably diverse and dynamic, with both acute and chronic dietary exposures significantly affecting the overall microbial community. There has been a long-standing understanding of the contribution of dysbiosis (abnormal changes in intestinal microbiota composition) to the pathogenesis of some diseases of altered intestinal health. **The gut microbial ecosystem is arguably the largest endocrine organ in the body, capable of producing a wide range of biologically active compounds that, like hormones, may be carried in the circulation and distributed to distant sites within the host, thereby influencing different essential biological processes**. Gut microbial communities differ in vegetarians and vegans compared with omnivores. Gut microbiota serve as a filter for our largest environmental exposure-what we eat. Technically speaking, food is a foreign object that we take into our bodies in kilogram quantities every day. The microbial community within each of us significantly influences how we experience a meal. **Differences in gut microbiota composition are associated with the development of complex metabolic disorders such as obesity and insulin resistance** (Wen, et al., 2011).

Gut microbiome and metabolic syndrome.

The human intestine contains up to 1000 different species of bacteria, yeasts, and parasites, weighting approximately 2 kg and carrying at least 100 times as many genes as the whole human genome. This microbiological population renews itself every 3 days and has an active biomass of a major human organ. It is estimated that around 20-25% of the world's population has metabolic syndrome, and people are twice as likely to die from and three times as likely to have a heart attack or stroke compared with people without the syndrome. The gut microbiota is an important environmental factor involved in the regulation of body weight and energy homeostasis. One hypothesis is obese and lean individuals have distinct different microbiota with measurable differences in their ability to extract energy from their diet and to store it in fat tissue. Microbiota alteration by using pro- and prebiotic dietary supplements is a potential nutritional target in the management of obesity and obesity-related disorders. A probiotic is described typically as a bacterial supplement consisting of Lactobacillus acidophilus, Lactobacillus casei, and bifidobacteria. Prebiotics are fiber compounds that pass undigested and feed the gut microbiota that colonize the large intestine. There is increasing evidence that the gut microbiota plays a significant role in glucose homeostasis, the development of impaired fasting glucose, type 2 diabetes, and insulin resistance. The anti-inflammatory function of probiotics assists in treating low grade inflammation. Modification of intestinal microbiota by probiotics may have a role in the maintenance of a healthier gut microbiota and could be a potential adjuvant in the treatment of insulin resistance and type 2 diabetes. Several studies suggest that oral probiotics have useful effects on total cholesterol and LDL cholesterol for subjects with high, borderline, and normal cholesterol levels (Mazidi, Rezaie, Kengne, Mobarhan, & Ferns, 2016).

Women and testosterone

TESTOSTERONE IS GENERALLY ASSOCIATED WITH men, for obvious reasons. What many people overlook is the importance of testosterone in the female body as well. The most common endocrine disorder in women of childbearing age is polycystic ovarian syndrome with hyperadrogenism being one of the three criteria used to help define (requires 2 out of three criteria). We also fail to recognize that heart disease is more common in women than men. The relationship of testosterone and heart disease in women is an area with a lot of unanswered questions. Women with PCOS have a tremendous risk factor profile but seem to have a hormonal balance that protects them for a while from cardiovascular disease.

Testosterone in women-the clinical significance.

Testosterone is an essential hormone for women. It acts directly as an androgen in addition to being an obligatory precursor for biosynthesis of estradiol. **Control of testosterone production in women is not well understood because no feedback loop governing its production has been described.** At physiological concentrations, testosterone has favorable effects on vasomotor tone, endothelial function, and peripheral vascular resistance. **Low concentrations of endogenous total testosterone and**

bioavailable testosterone have an adverse effect on the risk of cardiovascular disease and a 2015 study suggested an adverse effect on the risk of cardiovascular disease with endogenous testosterone levels above the 95th percentile. Overall, the available observational data suggest that low concentrations of total, free, bioavailable testosterone, SHBG, and extremely high concentrations of endogenous bioavailable T are associated with a greater likelihood of atherosclerotic carotid disease, cardiovascular events, and total mortality. A hallmark of polycystic ovary syndrome is low concentrations of SHBG, which, in turn, are associated with the higher risk profile for cardiovascular disease. **Low concentrations of SHBG are an independent risk factor for insulin resistance, type 2 diabetes, and adverse lipid profile in young women and women at midlife.** Strong independent and highly significant inverse associations between insulin resistance and SHBG and between BMI and SHBG have been shown. These associations are independent of endogenous estrogen and androgen concentrations. **As SHBG levels decrease insulin resistance and BMI increase.**

Findings from basic studies have shown that estradiol and testosterone are neuroprotective and have anti-inflammatory actions within the brain. Concentrations of testosterone in the human female brain during the reproductive years are several times greater than concentrations of estradiol. Testosterone within the brain is protective against oxidative stress, apoptosis (cell death), and soluble amyloid B toxicity.

In the Women's Health Initiative observational study, higher concentrations of endogenous bioavailable testosterone were associated with lower occurrences of hip fracture independent of concentrations of estradiol and SHBG. **No randomized controlled trials have been reported on the effect of treatment with testosterone on fracture in women.** High concentrations of endogenous free testosterone have been directly associated with greater lean body mass in women aged 67-94 years old. Randomized controlled trials have shown greater increases in lean body mass and strength and greater reduction in percentage of fat in postmenopausal women given combined estrogen and testosterone compared with estrogen alone.

High endogenous concentrations of total testosterone, androstenedione, DHEAS, total and free estradiol, estrone were each independently associated with an increased risk of breast cancer but free testosterone was not. No reported clinical trial has been of sufficient duration to provide certainty about the safety of exogenous testosterone in terms of breast cancer, such that the effects of long-term use remain uncertain.

Adverse cardiovascular effects have not been seen in studies of transdermal testosterone therapy in women.

Many randomized placebo-controlled trials have shown that testosterone therapy can be effective in the treatment of female sexual dysfunction. Maximum concentrations of testosterone are achieved in the third and fourth decades, followed by a steady decline in testosterone and its precursors with increasing age. **Sexual function is not related to changes in circulating concentrations of androgens at menopause or early post-menopause, as blood concentrations of androgens do not change during the menopausal transition. The Endocrine Soci-**

ety has concluded "Evidence supports the short-term efficacy and safety of high physiological doses of testosterone treatment of post-menopausal women with sexual dysfunction due to hypoactive sexual desire disorder". (Davis & Wahlin-Jacobsen, 2015)

Sex differences in cardiovascular risk factors and disease prevention.

Abstract

Cardiovascular disease (CVD) has been seen as a men's disease for decades, however it is more common in women than in men. It is assumed in that the major risk factors (RF) on CVD outcomes are the same in women as in men. Common disorders of pregnancy, such as gestational hypertension, diabetes, as well as polycystic ovary syndrome (PCOS) and early menopause are associated with accelerated development of CVD. Furthermore, female-specific RFs might be identified enabling early detection of apparently healthy women with a high lifetime risk of CVD. A literature search was performed to examine the impact of female-specific RFs on the traditional RFs and the occurrence of CVD. We found that the effects of elevated blood pressure, overweight and obesity, and elevated cholesterol on CVD outcomes are largely similar between women and men, however **prolonged smoking is significantly more hazardous for women than for men**. With respect to female-specific RF only associations (and no absolute risk data) could be found between preeclampsia, gestational diabetes and menopause onset with the occurrence of CVD. This review shows that CVD is the main cause of death in men and women, however the prevalence is higher in women. There are differences in impact of major CV RF leading to a worse outcome in women. Lifestyle interventions and awareness in women needs more consideration. Attention for female specific RF may enable early detection and intervention in apparently healthy women. (Appelman, et al., 2015)

Low testosterone levels predict all-causes mortality and cardiovascular events in women: a prospective cohort study in German primary care patients.

The objective was to determine whether baseline testosterone levels in women are associated with future overall or CV morbidity and mortality. 2,914 female patients from German primary care practices with mean age of 57.96 years old and BMI 26.71 were followed for 4.5 years. **Women with total testosterone levels in the lowest quintile had a higher risk to die of any cause or to develop a CV event within the follow-up period compared to patients in the other quintiles independent of traditional risk factors** (Sievers, et al., 2010).

Androgen therapy in women: a reappraisal: An Endocrine Society clinical practice guideline.

1. Recommend against making a diagnosis of androgen deficiency syndrome in healthy women because there is a lack of a well-defined syndrome, and data correlating androgen levels with specific signs or symptoms are unavailable.

2. Recommend against the general use of T except for hypoactive sexual desire disorder.
3. Recommend against the routine prescription of T in women with low androgen levels.
4. Evidence supports the short-term efficacy and safety of high physiological doses of T treatment of postmenopausal women with sexual dysfunction due to hypoactive sexual desire disorder (Wierman, et al., 2014).

Clinical review: The benefits and harms of systemic testosterone therapy in postmenopausal women with normal adrenal function: a systematic review and meta-analysis.

The use of T has been suggested to improve women's health during the postmenopausal period. 35 randomized trials (5,053 women) were reviewed.

T use was associated with reduction in total cholesterol, triglyceride, HDL and increase in LDL, acne and hirsutism. A statistically significant improvement in various domains of sexual function. No significant effect was noted on anthropometric measures and bone density. Conclusion: despite the improvement in sexual function associated with T use in postmenopausal women, long-term safety data are lacking (Elraiyah, et al., 2014).

Reduced breast cancer incidence in women treated with subcutaneous testosterone, or testosterone with anastrozole: A prospective, observational study.

Excluding skin cancer, breast cancer is the most common cancer among women, with a lifetime risk of 1 in 8. It is well recognized that estrogen and progestin therapy stimulates breast tissue and increases the incidence of breast cancer. There is evidence that androgens are breast protective and that testosterone therapy treats many symptoms of hormone deficiency in both premenopausal and postmenopausal patients. **This study is a 5-year interim analysis of a 10-year study designed to investigate the incidence of breast cancer in women treated with subcutaneous testosterone therapy or testosterone/anastrozole therapy in the absence of systemic estrogen therapy.** There are many ways to treat symptoms and one approach is subcutaneous testosterone implants. Testosterone implants are made by a compound pharmacy and placed in the subcutaneous tissue approximately every 3 months and usually have 60 mg testosterone. Testosterone levels were not drawn on all patients and dosing was based on past experience using this approach. A concern is that T is the major substrate for estradiol and therefore has a secondary "stimulatory" effect at the estrogen receptor. Anastrozole, combined with T in a pellet implant, has been shown to prevent aromatization and provides adequate levels of T without elevating estradiol. Also, T has been shown to safely relieve side effects of aromatase inhibitor therapy (anastrozole) in breast cancer survivors.

The present data shows a remarkable lower breast cancer rate using subcutaneous testosterone with or without anastrozole when compared to all previous studies concerning hormonal treatments.

Androgens, including T pellet implants, have been used to successfully treat breast cancer in the past as well as symptoms of menopause in breast cancer survivors (Glaser & Dimitrakakis, 2013).

Cardiometabolic Aspects of the Polycystic Ovary Syndrome

Polycystic ovary syndrome (PCOS) is the most common endocrine disorder among women of reproductive age with a prevalence rate of between 5-10%. In general, women live longer than men and develop cardiovascular disease at an older age. The diagnostic criteria for PCOS requires two out of three abnormalities:

1. Oligo- or anovulation.
2. Clinical and/or biochemical signs of **hyper-androgenism** (excluding other diseases first).
3. Polycystic ovaries.

Women with PCOS have an increased prevalence of sleep apnea, insulin resistance, prediabetes, gestational diabetes, diabetes, atherogenic lipid profile, adipose-derived proinflammatory factors including CRP, obesity, android type obesity, increased prothrombotic state with increased spontaneous abortions, hypertension and decreased adiponectin values (anti-inflammatory factor) compared with age and BMI matched women without the syndrome.

Dyslipidemia is the most common abnormality in PCOS. The lipid pattern in women with PCOS is only modestly more atherogenic compared with control women with similar BMI.

The prevalence of OSA in women with PCOS compared to women without PCOS after adjustment for age and BMI is 5-to 30-fold higher.

More recently, Shaw et al (2008) evaluated the risk of cardiovascular events in 390 postmenopausal women enrolled in the NIH-National Heart, Lung, and Blood Institute-sponsored Women's Ischemia Syndrome Evaluation (WISE) study. Of the 390 women enrolled, a total of 104 women had PCOS. Interestingly, the authors reported that women with clinical features of PCOS had more angiographic coronary artery disease compared with women without clinical features of PCOS. The cumulative 5-yr cardiovascular event-free survival was 78.9% for women with PCOS vs. 88.7% for women without clinical features of PCOS. The 2-fold increase in cardiac events in the PCOS women is similar to the 2-fold increased risk of a fatal myocardial infarction in PCOS women reported in a 2002 study. The average age of the women in the WISE study was 63 years old, and the cardiovascular event-free survival curves diverged immediately from entry into the study, suggesting that cardiovascular events may occur at an earlier age in PCOS women compared with normal women.

Perhaps the best quality data is from the Nurse's Health Study. Putting it all together, the "absolute" risk for vascular events for most women with PCOS will remain relatively low due to both young age and female gender.

The most extensively studied insulin lowering drug in the treatment of PCOS is metformin. Metformin reduced blood pressure, fasting glucose, and serum androgens with no effect on body weight or hirsutism scores. Metformin improves metabolic parameters in PCOS women. **A meta-analysis that included 14 trials with PCOS subjects demonstrated a decrease by 40% of new-onset DM and a reduction by 6% in the absolute risk of DM with metformin.** (Randeva, et al., 2012)

Mortality of women with polycystic ovary syndrome at long-term follow-up.

Metabolic disturbances associated with insulin resistance are present in most women with polycystic ovary syndrome. This has led to suggestions that women with PCOS may be at increased risk of cardiovascular disease in later life. A total of 786 women diagnosed with PCOS in England between 1930 and 1979 were traced from hospital records and followed for an average of 30 years.

Women with PCOS did not have markedly higher than average mortality from circulatory disease, even though the condition is strongly associated with diabetes, lipid abnormalities, and other cardiovascular risk factors (Pierpoint, McKeigue, Isaacs, Wild, & Jacobs, 1998).

Cardiovascular disease in women with polycystic ovary syndrome at long-term follow-up: a retrospective cohort study.

Morbidity data were collected from 319 women with PCOS and 1,060 age-matched control women. All-cause and cardiovascular mortality were similar in women with PCOS compared with control women. A history of coronary heart disease was not significantly more common in women with PCOS but the odds ratio for nonfatal cerebrovascular disease was 2.8. **Morbidity and mortality from coronary heart disease was not higher compared to the general public despite higher levels of cardiovascular risk factors in PCOS women** (Wild, Pierpoint, McKeigue, & Jacobs, 2000).

Prevalence of 'obesity-associated gonadal dysfunction' in severely obese men and women and its resolution after bariatric surgery: a systematic review and meta-analysis.

Abstract

BACKGROUND:

Sexual dimorphism manifests noticeably in obesity-associated gonadal dysfunction. In women, obesity is associated with androgen excess disorders, mostly polycystic ovary syndrome (PCOS), whereas androgen deficiency is frequently present in obese men in what has been termed as male obesity-associated secondary hypogonadism (MOSH).

OBJECTIVE AND RATIONALE:

We aimed to obtain an estimation of the prevalence of obesity-associated gonadal dysfunction among women and men presenting with severe obesity and to evaluate the response to bariatric surgery and changes in circulating sex hormone concentrations.

OUTCOMES:

In severely obese patients submitted to bariatric surgery, obesity-associated gonadal dysfunction was very prevalent: PCOS was present in 36% (95CI 22-50) of women and MOSH was present in 64% (95CI 50-77) of men. After bariatric surgery, resolution of PCOS was found in 96% (95CI 89-100) of affected women and resolution of MOSH occurred in 87% of affected men. Sex hormone-binding globulin concentrations increased after bariatric surgery in women and in men and serum estradiol concentrations decreased in women and to a lesser extent in men. On the contrary, sex-specific changes were observed in serum androgen concentrations: for example, total testosterone concentration increased in men but decreased in women. The latter was accompanied by resolution of hirsutism in 53%, and of menstrual dysfunction in 96%, of women showing these symptoms before surgery.

WIDER IMPLICATIONS:

Obesity-associated gonadal dysfunction is among the most prevalent comorbidities in patients with severe obesity and should be ruled out routinely during their initial diagnostic workup. Considering the excellent response regarding both PCOS and MOSH, bariatric surgery should be offered to severely obese patients presenting with obesity-associated gonadal dysfunction (Escobar-Morreale, Santacruz, Luque-Ramírez, & Botella Carretero, 2017)

Evidence not supporting testosterone

FOUR ARTICLES (FINKLE 2014, VIGEN 2013, Basaria 2010, and Xu 2013) have complicated the relationship between Testosterone and heart disease. In January 2014, the US FDA announced plans to review the possibility that testosterone products increase the risk of adverse cardiovascular events based on the Finkle and Vigen studies below.

Increased risk of non-fatal myocardial infarction following testosterone therapy prescription in men.

> The study analyzed health insurance data involving diagnosis codes and prescriptions, and reported that men who received a testosterone script had a greater risk of nonfatal heart attack in the next 90 days than in the prior 12 months compared to men who did not receive any script. The actual increased risk was just over 1 event for every 1,000 years of Testosterone use (Finkle, et al., 2014).

Association of testosterone therapy with mortality, myocardial infarction, and stroke in men with low testosterone levels.

> The authors concluded that more cardiac events occurred in the testosterone treated group compared to the

non-testosterone treated group. 29 medical societies have called for retraction of the study, citing "gross data mismanagement and contamination" rendering the study "no longer credible" The percentage of men who suffered an event was lower by one half for the T group compared to the non-T group when the raw data was reviewed. (10.1% in T group vs 21.2% in non-T group). The authors improperly excluded 1132 men and even had 10% women included inappropriately. Also, an event in the T-group was given more "weight" than the same event in the untreated arm (Vigen, et al., 2013).

Adverse events associated with testosterone administration.

Reported an increase in CV-related symptoms or events. Study used twice the standard routine clinical initiation dose of testosterone in frail elderly men with a high number of co-morbidities. Study counted symptoms such as edema, palpitations as events which is usually not the standard (Basaria, et al., 2010).

Testosterone therapy and cardiovascular events among men. A systematic review and meta-analysis of placebo-controlled randomized trials.

Authors assessed CV events in 27 placebo-controlled studies of 12-weeks duration or longer and reported CV events were greater in the men who received T compared with placebo. The problem with the meta-analysis was two of the 27 studies contributed 35 % of all CV events. One of the studies was the Basaria study above and the other study gave oral T at very high doses (600 mg) to cirrhotic patients. Oral T promotes liver disease especially at toxic doses to men with cirrhosis. **This study provided no relevant information.** Without these two studies, the rates of adverse CV events were similar, with a slightly lower rate in the T group (Xu, Freeman, Cowling, & Schooling, 2013)

Negative effects with testosterone usage include:

1. Increases platelet thromboxane A2 receptor density and platelet aggregation-potentially thrombogenic.
2. Decreased sperm production and testicle size.
3. Swelling/tenderness of breasts, swelling of feet and ankles.
4. Worsen obstructive sleep apnea by inhibiting hypercapnic respiratory drive (Xu, Freeman, Cowling, & Schooling, 2013).

Hypogonadism in Elderly Men- What to Do Until the Evidence Comes

The serum total testosterone concentration decreases from a mean of about 600 ng per deciliter at 30 years of age to a mean of about 400 ng per deciliter at 80 years, although the range is wide at all ages. An essential but still unanswered question is whether this decrease in the testosterone concentration is physiologic, perhaps conveying a benefit, or pathologic, causing harm. According to one estimate, a study would need to include 6000 elderly hypogonadal men randomly assigned to receive testosterone or placebo for six years to determine whether testosterone treatment increases the risk of prostate cancer by 30 percent. Difficult questions require large numbers of participants over a long duration of time and many times the studies will never be done for practical or financial reasons. With data over the last 13 years, we can comfortably say that low testosterone has negative consequences on many systems of the body and is a biomarker of illness. This was written 13 years ago and the evidence is present now (Snyder P. , 2004).

Clinical Meaningfulness of the Changes in Muscle Performance and Physical and Function Associated with Testosterone Administration In Older Men With Mobility Limitation.

Men aged 65 years and older, with mobility limitations, with total T levels 100-350 ng/dl were randomized to placebo or 10 grams T gel daily for 6 months in a parallel group, double-blind trial. Mobility limitations were defined as difficulty walking two blocks or climbing 10 steps. T dose could be increased or decreased based on T levels and 106 men received T gel and 103 men received a placebo gel. The mean age was 74 years old. Leg -press strength was one of measures studied since it is an important component in walking and climbing stairs. **The study was halted after enrolling 209 of the planned 252 patients over a three-year period because 23 patients in the treatment group vs 5 in the placebo had adverse cardiovascular events. The specific cardiovascular events were not defined.** The men assigned to the testosterone arm experienced greater gains in leg-press strength, chest-press strength and power, skeletal muscle mass and loaded stair-climbing power. Walking speed, a key determinant of mobility, did not change significantly. **The improvements in muscle mass and strength need to be weighed against the greater risk of adverse cardiovascular events in the testosterone gel group** (Travison, et al., 2011). Remember, topical testosterone increases DHT levels more than shots and this could be the potential answer.

Treatment of Men for "Low Testosterone": A Systematic Review.

A systematic review of randomized controlled trials involving "low testosterone" for cardiovascular health, sexual function, muscle weakness or wasting, mood and behavior, and cognition conducted by several members that included a watchdog group named Pharmed Out at Georgetown University that promotes evidence based prescribing. **Despite several studies reviewed showing positive benefits, the summary statement felt that testosterone supplementation for "low T" for cardiovascular health, sexual function, physical function, mood, or cognitive function is without support from randomized clinical trials.**

Based on my reviewing some of the same articles, there seemed to be bias and lack of intellectual rigor in analyzing many of the articles. Broad generalizations are made which only cloud the many questions involving testosterone treatment (Huo, et al., 2016).

In 2004, the Institute of Medicine reviewed the evidence on T therapy and concluded "there is not clear evidence of benefit for any of the health outcomes examined." (Institute of Medicine (US) Committee on Assessing the Need for Clinical Trials, 2004). This is 13 years ago.

T therapy in older men is done on a case by case basis with explicit discussion of the uncertainty about the risks and benefits of T therapy. For example, men receiving high dose glucocorticoids who have low T levels can help preserve bone mass and bone mineral density with T therapy. Administration of more than 5-7.5 mg/day of prednisone or its equivalent increases the risk of gonadotropin and T suppression and alterations in muscle and bone mass.

Clinical trials on the effects of T on cognitive function have revealed inconclusive results. The current evidence is insufficient to conclude that T therapy is beneficial or harmful to cognitive function. The effects of T on depression have also been inconsistent.

Endocrine Society Clinical Practice Guidelines 2010.

An evaluation of androgen deficiency should not be made during an acute or subacute illness. We recommend against screening for androgen deficiency in the general population. In men receiving T shots we suggest aiming for T levels between 400-700 one week after injection. If hematocrit is above 54%, stop therapy until hematocrit decreases to a safer level, evaluate the patient for hypoxia and sleep apnea and reinitiate therapy at a reduced dose. **The frequency of neuro-occlusive events (CVA) in association with increased hematocrit in T trials has been extremely low. We recommend against a general policy of offering T therapy to all older men with low T levels.**

The Endocrine Society recommends against T therapy in pts who desire fertility (endogenous T downregulates LH/spermatogenesis).

Surprisingly, recent evidence suggests that anabolic steroid use may be the most common cause of hypogonadism in men of reproductive age.

In trials funded by the pharmaceutical industry testosterone had no effect on cardiovascular-related events, but in non-funded trials testosterone therapy substantially increased the risk of a CV-related event. 33 CV related deaths were identified (22 T arm, 11 placebo arm). T therapy increases CV-related events among men. The studies that support the cardiac safety of testosterone greatly outweigh the studies that say the opposite.

Testosterone stimulates hepatic lipase activity which in turn has been shown to decrease HDL-C and LDL particle size and thus results in a more atherogenic lipid profile.

Testosterone therapy and risk of myocardial infarction: a pharmacoepidemiological study.

A case-control study within a cohort of 934,283 men aged 45-80 years old from a health claim database were studied looking for a relationship between myocardial infarction and testosterone replacement therapy. 30,066 MI cases with 120,264 corresponding controls were studied. **Current use of testosterone was not associated with an increased risk of MI. First time users did show an increased risk, although the absolute risk was low (number needed to harm 301). First time users usually have more cardiac risk factors and have not taken testosterone long enough to provide any benefit. A** study of Intramuscular T (200 mg every 2 weeks for 36 months) demonstrated a larger increase in fat-free mass (6.7%) and a larger decrease in the proportion of body fat (17.3%). Although a pharmacologic dose of T may have a marked effect on body composition and function, low-dose replacement consisting of 75 mg daily DHEA or 5 mg T patch had no demonstrable effect. Our data provide no evidence that either DHEA or low-dose T is an effective anti-aging hormone supplement and argue strongly against the use of these agents for this purpose (Etminan, Skeldon, Goldenberg, Carleton, & Brophy, 2015).

Risk and benefits of testosterone therapy in older men.

The age-related decline in testosterone levels is caused by defects at all levels of the hypothalamic-pituitary-testicular axis, and the trajectory of decline is affected by BMI, weight gain, comorbid conditions, medications and genetic factors. By combining symptoms, total testosterone, and sometimes LH levels, the diagnostic accuracy of hypogonadism may improve. The review repeats many common held principles about testosterone.

Testosterone levels are not significantly associated with lower urinary tract symptoms, ageing-related psychological symptoms and erectile function.

The association of testosterone with measures of depression and cognition has been inconsistent. Current evidence is insufficient to conclude that testosterone therapy is beneficial or harmful to cognitive function.

Androgen deficiency and erectile dysfunction are two distinct syndromes that are independently distributed in men. Randomized trials have failed to support the hypothesis that addition of testosterone to PDE5I (phosphodiesterase type 5 inhibitors – Viagra, Cialis, etc.) improves erectile dysfunction. Clinically we may give T therapy to improve erectile dysfunction but we need to express that this may or may not be helpful. Erectile dysfunction is complicated and can be the first symptom of cardiovascular disease. Testosterone has also been reported to increase muscle protein synthesis and reduce protein degradation. A meta-analysis revealed that testosterone therapy is associated with an average 0.8 g/dl increase in hemoglobin. The Endocrine Society's expert panel recommends that testosterone administration should be withheld in men whose Hematocrit rises above 54% during testosterone therapy. Testosterone administration depresses hypercapnic ventilator drive, thus may aggravate OSA. The average increase in PSA levels with testosterone therapy in healthy men with hypogonadism is 0.30 ng/ml in young and 0.43 ng/ml in older men (Spitzer, Huang, Basaria, Travison, & Bhasin, 2013).

Extremes of Endogenous Testosterone Are Associated with Increased Risk of Incident Coronary Events in Older Women.

Prospective, population-based study of 639 healthy non-estrogen-using postmenopausal women, aged 50-91 (mean 73.8) years old had baseline serum T levels followed for a median time of 12.3 years (20 years total period) for incident cardiovascular events (nonfatal MI, fatal MI, and coronary revascularizations). During a median follow-up of 12.3 years, 134 women has a first CHD event; 45 were nonfatal MIs, 10 were coronary revascularizations, and

79 were CHD deaths. The lowest total T quintile (lowest 20%) was associated with a 62% increased risk of incident CHD. **Bioavailable T showed a U-shaped association with incident CHD. The lowest 20% levels and highest 20% Bio-T levels showed a 79% and 96% increased risk compared to the other quintiles.** These results were not explained by age, adiposity, lifestyle, or ovarian status. In this and other studies, higher levels of endogenous BioT in postmenopausal women are associated with adiposity and adiposity-related conditions including higher BMI, larger waist girth, insulin resistance, adverse lipid profiles, type 2 diabetes, and the metabolic syndrome.

It is not clear whether high BioT is a marker or a mediator of CHD risk.

Conclusion- An optimal range of testosterone may exist for cardiovascular health in women, with increased risk of CHD events at low levels of testosterone and at high levels of Bio-T.

Natural experiments suggest that lower lifetime endogenous androgens (men with Klinefelter syndrome and legally castrated men) are associated with a relatively lower risk of death from ischemic heart disease. This contradicts the data supporting low T as a risk factor for ischemic heart disease. (Laughlin, Goodell, & Barrett-Connor, 2010)

Testosterone use in men and its effects on bone health. A systematic review and meta-analysis of randomized placebo-controlled trials.

Androgen-deficient men are at increased risk of osteoporosis. We performed a systematic review and meta-analysis of randomized placebo-controlled trials in men to estimate the effect of testosterone use on bone health outcomes. We included eight trials enrolling 365 patients. Two trials followed patients for more than one year.

IM testosterone - 8% increase in lumbar bone density, 4% increase in femoral density compared to placebo.

Topical testosterone (gel) had no significant impact.

No bone fracture data noted, therefore this study provides only indirect potential about clinical utility of testosterone on treatment/prevention of osteoporosis (Tracz, et al., 2006).

In healthy middle-aged men T does not predict cardiovascular disease. In elderly men (over 70) low T predicts increased cardiovascular disease and/or mortality. It is at present unclear whether low T has a direct negative effect, or whether it should be regarded as a 'marker of poor health'. Recent studies on T and CVD/mortality show more pronounced associations than earlier studies.

Testosterone and Male Infertility

Infertility is the inability to conceive after 12 months of unprotected intercourse. Approximately 15% of couples have infertility, but only 20% seek evaluation. In 30%, a significant male factor is responsible. An additional 20% of couples have both male and female factors, thus male factors contribute to 50% to infertile situations. **Exogenous testosterone is a known and common cause of infertility in men. Exogenous testosterone should be** discontinued in any male trying to achieve pregnancy (Ohlander, Lindgren, & Lipshultz, 2016).

Prevalence of 'obesity-associated gonadal dysfunction' in severely obese men and women and its resolution after bariatric surgery: a systematic review and meta-analysis.

Abstract
BACKGROUND:
Sexual dimorphism manifests noticeably in obesity-associated gonadal dysfunction. In women, obesity is associated with androgen excess disorders, mostly polycystic ovary syndrome (PCOS), whereas androgen deficiency is frequently present in obese men in what has been termed as male obesity-associated secondary hypogonadism (MOSH).

OBJECTIVE AND RATIONALE:
We aimed to obtain an estimation of the prevalence of obesity-associated gonadal dysfunction among women and men presenting with severe obesity and to evaluate the response to bariatric surgery and changes in circulating sex hormone concentrations.

OUTCOMES:
In severely obese patients submitted to bariatric surgery, obesity-associated gonadal dysfunction was very prevalent: PCOS was present in 36% (95CI 22-50) of women and MOSH was present in 64% (95CI 50-77) of men. After bariatric surgery, resolution of PCOS was found in 96% (95CI 89-100) of affected women and resolution of MOSH occurred in 87% of affected men. Sex hormone-binding globulin concentrations increased after bariatric surgery

in women and in men and serum estradiol concentrations decreased in women and to a lesser extent in men. On the contrary, sex-specific changes were observed in serum androgen concentrations: for example, total testosterone concentration increased in men but decreased in women. The latter was accompanied by resolution of hirsutism in 53%, and of menstrual dysfunction in 96%, of women showing these symptoms before surgery.

WIDER IMPLICATIONS: Obesity-associated gonadal dysfunction is among the most prevalent comorbidities in patients with severe obesity and should be ruled out routinely during their initial diagnostic workup. Considering the excellent response regarding both PCOS and MOSH, bariatric surgery should be offered to severely obese patients presenting with obesity-associated gonadal dysfunction (Escobar-Morreale, Santacruz, Luque-Ramírez, & Botella Carretero, 2017).

Conclusion

I HAVE TRIED TO SELECT articles with good science behind them along with interesting ideas and lessons to learn from. I have tried to be balanced to allow the reader to come to their own conclusions.

Minorities need to be included for better understanding. I have great admiration towards the researchers and clinicians that asked the important questions in their articles

References

Abdullah, S., Barkley, K., Bhella, P., Hastings, J., Matulevicius, S., Fujimoto, N., . . . Levine, B. (2016). Lifelong Physical Activity Regardless of Dose Is Not Associated with Myocardial Fibrosis. *Circulation: Cardiovascular Imaging, 9*. doi:https://doi.org/10.1161/CIRCIMAGING.116.005511

Ahlskog, J., Geda, Y., Graff-Radford, N., & Petersen, R. (2011, Sept). Physical exercise as a preventive or disease-modifying treatment of dementia and brain aging. *Mayo Clinic Proceedings, 86*(9), 876-84. doi:https://doi.org/10.4065/mcp.2011.0252

Albertson, T., Chenoweth, J., Colby, D., & Sutter, M. (2016). The Changing Drug Culture: Use and Misuse of Appearance- and Performance-Enhancing Drugs. *FP Essentials, 441*, 30-43.

Allan, C., Strauss, B., Forbes, E., Paul, E., & McLachlan, R. (2011). Variability in total testosterone levels in ageing men with symptoms of androgen deficiency. *International Journal of Andrology, 34*(3), 212-216. doi:https://doi.org/10.1111/j.1365-2605.2010.01071.x

Amory, J., Chansky, H., Chansky, K., Camuso, M., Hoey, C., Anawalt, B., . . . Bremner, W. (2002). Preoperative Supraphysiological Testosterone in Older Men Undergoing Knee Replacement Surgery. *Journal of the American*

Geriatrics Society, 50(10), 1698-1701. doi:10.1046/j.1532-5415.2002.50462.x

Andreassen, M., Raymond, I., Kistorp, C., Hildebrandt, P., Faber, J., & Kristensen, L. (2009). IGF1 as predictor of all-cause mortality and cardiovascular disease in an elderly population. *European Journal of Endocrinology, 160*(1), 25-31. doi:https://doi.org/10.1530/EJE-08-0452

Appelman, Y., Rijn, v., BB, Ten Haaf, M., Boersma, E., & Peters, S. (2015). Sex differences in cardiovascular risk factors and disease prevention. *Atherosclerosis, 241*(1), 211-8. doi:https://doi.org/10.1016/j.atherosclerosis.2015.01.027

Araujo, A., Dixon, J., Suarez, E., Murad, M., Guey, L., & Wittert, G. (2011). Clinical review: Endogenous testosterone and mortality in men: a systematic review and meta-analysis. *The Journal of Clinical Endocrinology and Metabolism, 96*(10), 3007-3019. doi:https://doi.org/10.1210/jc.2011-1137

Arnett, S., Laity, J., Agrawal, S., & Cress, M. (2008). Aerobic reserve and physical functional performance in older adults. *Age and Ageing, 37*(4), 384-9. doi:https://doi.org/10.1093/ageing/afn022

Atkinson, R., Srinivas-Shankar, U., Roberts, S., Connolly, M., Adams, J., Oldham, J., . . . Narici, M. (2010). Effects of Testosterone on Skeletal Muscle Architecture in Intermediate-Frail and Frail Elderly Men. *J Gerontol A Biol Sci Med Sci, 65a*(11), 1215-1219. doi:https://doi.org/10.1093/gerona/glq118

Baas, W., & Köhler, T. (2016). Testosterone replacement therapy and voiding dysfunction. *Translational Andrology and Urology, 5*(6), 890-897. doi:https://dx.doi.org/10.21037%2Ftau.2016.08.11

REFERENCES

Baillargeon, J., Deer, R., Kuo, Y., Zhang, D., Goodwin, J., & Volpi, E. (2016). Androgen Therapy and Re-hospitalization in Older Men With Testosterone Deficiency. *Mayo Clinic Proceedings, 91*(5), 587-95. doi:https://doi.org/10.1016/j.mayocp.2016.03.016

Baillargeon, J., Urban, R., Kuo, Y., Ottenbacher, K., Raji, M., Du, F., . . . Goodwin, J. (2014). Risk of Myocardial Infarction in Older Men Receiving Testosterone Therapy. *Annals of Pharmacotherapy, 48*(9), 1138-1144. doi:https://doi.org/10.1177/1060028014539918

Bann, D., Hire, D., Manini, T., Cooper, R., Botoseneanu, A., McDermott, M., . . . Group, L. S. (2013, Feb 3). Light Intensity physical activity and sedentary behavior in relation to body mass index and grip strength in older adults: cross-sectional findings from the Lifestyle Interventions and Independence for Elders (LIFE) study. *Plos one, 10*(2). doi:https://doi.org/10.1371/journal.pone.0116058

Basaria, S., Coviello, A., Travison, T., Storer, T., Farwell, W., Jette, A., . . . Aggarwal, S. (2010). Adverse events associated with testosterone administration. *New England Journal of Medicine, 363*(2), 109-22. doi:https://doi.org/10.1056/NEJMoa1000485

Bauman, W., La Fountaine, M., Cirnigliaro, C., Kirshblum, S., & Spungen, A. (2015). Lean tissue mass and energy expenditure are retained in hypogonadal men with spinal cord injury after discontinuation of testosterone replacement therapy. *The Journal of Spinal Cord Medicine, 38*(1), 38-47. doi:https://doi.org/10.1179/2045772314Y.0000000206

Bhasin, S., Woodhouse, L., Casaburi, R., Singh, A., Bhasin, D., Berman, N., . . . Storer, T. (2001). Testosterone dose-response relationships in healthy young men. *The American Journal* of *Physiology, Endocrinology, and Metabolism, 281*(6). Retrieved from http://ajpendo.physiology.org/content/281/6/E1172.long

Bhasin, S., Woodhouse, L., Casaburi, R., Singh, A., Mac, R., Lee, M., . . . Storer, T. (2005). Older Men Are as Responsive as Young Men to the Anabolic Effects of Graded Doses of Testosterone on the Skeletal Muscle. *Journal of Clinical Endocrinology and Metabolism, 90*(2), 678-688. doi:https://doi.org/10.1210/jc.2004-1184

Bischoff-Ferrari, H., Orav, E., & Dawson-Hughes, B. (2008). Additive benefit of higher testosterone levels and vitamin D plus calcium supplementation in regard to fall risk reduction among older men and women. *Osteoporosis International, 19*(9), 1307-14. doi:https://doi.org/10.1007/s00198-008-0573-7

Blackman, M., Sorkin, J., Münzer, T., Bellantoni, M., Busby-Whitehead, J., Stevens, T., . . . Harman, S. (2002). Growth Hormone and Sex Steroid Administration in Healthy Aged Women and Men. A Randomized Controlled Trial. *JAMA, 288*(18), 2282-92. doi:10.1001/jama.288.18.2282

Boolell, M., Allen, M., Ballard, S., Gepi-Attee, S., Muirhead, G., Naylor, A., . . . Gingell, C. (1996). Sildenafil: an orally active type 5 cyclic GMP-specific phosphodiesterase inhibitor for the treatment of penile erectile dysfunction. *International Journal of Impotence Research, 8*(2), 47-52.

Boolell, M., Gepi-Attee, S., Gingell, J., & Allen, M. (1996). Sildenafil, a novel effective oral therapy for male erectile dysfunction. *British Journal of Urology, 78*(2), 257-61.

Borst, S., & Yarrow, J. (2015). Injection of testosterone may be safer and more effective than transdermal administration for combating loss of muscle and bone in older men. *The American Journal of Physiology. Endocrinology and Metabolism, 308*(12), e1035-1042. doi:https://doi.org/10.1152/ajpendo.00111.2015

Bowditch, M., & Villar, R. (1999). Do obese patients bleed more? A prospective study of blood loss at total hip replacement. *Annals of the Royal College of Surgeons of England, 81*(3), 198-200. Retrieved from https://www.researchgate.net/publication/12933968_Do_obese_patients_bleed_more_A_prospective_study_of_blood_loss_at_total_hip_replacement

Brambilla, D., Matsumoto, A., Araujo, A., & McKinlay, J. (2009). The Effect of Diurnal Variation on Clinical measurement of Serum Testosterone and Other Sex Hormone Levels in Men. *Journal of Clinical Endocrinology and Metabolism, 94*(3), 907-913. doi:https://doi.org/10.1210/jc.2008-1902

Brook, M., Wilkinson, D., Mitchell, W., Lund, J., Phillips, B., Szewczyk, N., . . . Atherton, P. (2016). Synchronous deficits in cumulative muscle protein synthesis and ribosomal biogenesis underlie age-related anabolic resistance to exercise in humans. *Journal of Physiology, 594*(24), 7399-7417. doi:https://dx.doi.org/10.1113%2FJP272857

Brooke, J., Walter, D., Kapoor, D., Marsh, H., Muraleedharan, V., & Jones, T. (2014). Testosterone deficiency and severity of erectile dysfunction are independently associated with reduced quality of life in men with type 2 diabetes. *Andrology, 2*(2), 205-211. doi:https://doi.org/10.1111/j.2047-2927.2013.00177.x

Buvat J, M. M. (2013). Testosterone Deficiency in Men: Systematic Review and Standard Operating Procedures for Diagnosis and Treatment. *Journal of Sexual Medicine, 10*(1), 245-284. doi:https://doi.org/10.1111/j.1743-6109.2012.02783.x

Candow, D., Vogt, E., Johannsmeyer, S., Forbes, S., & Farthing, J. (2015). Strategic creatine supplementation and resistance training in healthy older adults. *Applied Physiology, Nutrition, and Metabolism, 40*(7), 689-94. doi:https://doi.org/10.1139/apnm-2014-0498

Carling, M., Jeppsson, A., Eriksson, B., & Brisby, H. (2015). Transfusions and blood loss in total hip and knee arthroplasty: a prospective observational study. *Journal of Orthopaedic Surgery and Research, 10*(48). Retrieved from https://josr-online.biomedcentral.com/articles/10.1186/s13018-015-0188-6

Christou, G., Christou, K., Nikas, D., & Goudevenos, J. (2016). Acute myocardial infarction in a young bodybuilder taking anabolic androgenic steroids: A case report and critical review of the literature. *European Journal of Preventative Cardiology, 23*(16), 1785-1796. doi:https://doi.org/10.1177/2047487316651341

Christou, M., Christou, P., Markozannes, G., Tsatsoulis, A., Mastorakos, G., & Tigas, S. (2017). Effects of Anabolic Androgenic Steroids on the Reproductive System of Athletes and Recreational Users: A Systematic Review and Meta-Analysis. *Sports Medicine.* doi:https://doi.org/10.1007/s40279-017-0709-z

Corona, G., Maseroli, E., & Maggi, M. (2014). Injectable testosterone undecanoate for the treatment of hypogonadism. *Expert Oninion on Pharmacotherapy*, 1903-26.

Corona, G., Maseroli, E., Rastrelli, G., Isidori, A., Sforza, A., Mannucci, E., & Maggi, M. (2014). Cardiovascular risk associated with testosterone-boosting medications: a systematic review and meta-analysis. *Expert Opinions on Drug Safety, 13*(10), 1327-1351. doi:https://doi.org/10.1517/14740338.2014.950653

REFERENCES

Corona, G., Monami, M., Rastrelli, G., Aversa, A., Sforza, A., Lenzi, A., . . . Maggi, M. (2010). Type 2 diabetes mellitus and testosterone: a meta-analysis study. *International Journal of Andrology, 34*(6), 528-40. doi:https://doi.org/10.1111/j.1365-2605.2010.01117.x

Coto-Montes, A., Boga, J., Tan, D., & Reiter, R. (2016). Melatonin as a Potential Agent in the Treatment of Sarcopenia. *International Journal of Molecular Sciences, 17*(10), 1771. doi:https://doi.org/10.3390/ijms17101771

Crewther, B., Cook, C., Cardinale, M., Weatherby, R., & Lowe, T. (n.d.). Two Emerging Concepts for Elite Athletes. The Short-Term Effects of Testosterone and Cortisol on the Neuromuscular System and the Dose-Response Training Role of these Endogenous Hormones. *Sports Medicine, 41*(2), 103-123. doi:https://doi.org/10.2165/11539170-000000000-00000

Crewther, B., Cronin, J., Keogh, J., & Cook, C. (2008). The Salivary Testosterone and Cortisol Response to Three Loading Schemes. *Journal of Strength and Conditioning Research, 22*(1), 250-255. doi:https://doi.org/10.1519/JSC.0b013e31815f5f91

Cunningham, G., & Toma, S. (2011). Clinical review: Why is androgen replacement in males controversial? *The Journal of Clinical Endocrinology and Metabolism, 96*(1), 38-52. doi:https://doi.org/10.1210/jc.2010-0266

Daka, B., Langer, R., Larsson, C., Rosén, T., Jansson, P., Råstam, L., & Lindblad, U. (2015). Low concentrations of serum testosterone predict acute myocardial infarction in men with type 2 diabetes mellitus. *BMC Endocr Disord, 15*(35). doi:https://doi.org/10.1186/s12902-015-0034-1

Davis, S., & Wahlin-Jacobsen, S. (2015). Testosterone in women- the clinical significance. *The Lancet. Diabetes and Endo-

crinology, 3(12), 980-92. doi:https://doi.org/10.1016/S2213-8587(15)00284-3

Dev, R., Bruera, E., & Del Fabbro, E. (2014). When and when not to use testosterone for palliation in cancer care. *Current Oncology Reports, 16*(4), 378. doi:https://doi.org/10.1007/s11912-014-0378-0

Dev, R., Hui, D., Fabbro, D., E, Delgado-Guay, MO, . . . Bruera, E. (2014). The Association Among Hypogonadism, Symptom Burden, and Survival in Male Patients with Advanced Cancer. . *Cancer, 120*(10), 1586-1593. doi:https://dx.doi.org/10.1002%2Fcncr.28619

Dhindsa, S., Ghanim, H., Batra, M., Kuhadiya, N., Abuaysheh, S., Green, K., . . . Dandona, P. (2016). Effect of testosterone on hepcidin, ferroportin, ferritin, and iron binding capacity in patients with hypogonadotropic hypogonadism and type 2 diabetes. *Clinical Endocrinology, 85*(5), 772-780. doi:https://doi.org/10.1111/cen.13130

Dhindsa, S., Ghanim, H., Batra, M., Kuhadiya, N., Abuaysheh, S., Sandhu, S., . . . Dandona, P. (2016). Insulin Resistance and Inflammation in Hypogonadotropic Hypogonadism and Their Reduction After Testosterone Replacement in Men With Type 2 Diabetes. *Diabetes Care, 39*(1), 82-91. doi:https://doi.org/10.2337/dc15-1518

Dhindsa, S., Miller, M., McWhirter, C., Mager, D., Ghanim, H., Chaudhuri, A., & Dandona, P. (2010). Testosterone concentrations in diabetic and nondiabetic obese men. *Diabetes care, 33*(6), 1186-92. doi:https://doi.org/10.2337/dc09-1649

Dimitrakakis, C., & Bondy, C. (2009). Androgens and the breast. *Breast Cancer Research, 11*(5), 212. doi:https://dx.doi.org/10.1186%2Fbcr2413

REFERENCES

Ding, E., Song, Y., Malik, V., & Liu, S. (2006). Sex differences of endogenous sex hormones and risk of type 2 diabetes: a systematic review and meta-analysis. *JAMA, 295*(11), 1288-99. doi:https://doi.org/10.1001/jama.295.11.1288

Dunstan, D., Daly, R., Owen, N., Jolley, D., Vulikh, E., Shaw, J., & Zimmet, P. (2005, Jan). Home-based resistance training is not sufficient to maintain improved glycemic control following supervised training in older individuals with type 2 diabetes. *Diabetes Care, 28*(1), 3-9. doi:https://doi.org/10.2337/diacare.28.1.3

Elraiyah, T., Sonbol, M., Wang, Z., Khairalseed, T., Asi, N., Undavalli, C., . . . MH, M. (2014). Clinical review: The benefits and harms of systemic testosterone therapy in postmenopausal women with normal adrenal function: a systematic review and meta-analysis. *Journal of Clinical Endocrinology and Metabolism, 99*(10), 3543-50. doi:https://doi.org/10.1210/jc.2014-2262

English, K., Steeds, R., Jones, T., Diver, M., & Channer, K. (2000). Low-dose transdermal testosterone therapy improves angina threshold in men with chronic stable angina: A randomized, double-blind, placebo-controlled study. *Circulations, 102*(16), 1906-11. doi:https://doi.org/10.1161/01.CIR.102.16.1906

Escobar-Morreale, H., Santacruz, E., Luque-Ramírez, M., & Botella Carretero, J. (2017). Prevalence of 'obesity-associated gonadal dysfunction' in severely obese men and women and its resolution after bariatric surgery: a systematic review and meta-analysis. *Human Reproduction Update, 9*, 1-19. doi:https://doi.org/10.1093/humupd/dmx012

Etminan, M., Skeldon, S., Goldenberg, S., Carleton, B., & Brophy, J. (2015). Testosterone therapy and risk of myocardial infarction: a pharmacoepidemiological study. *Pharmacotherapy, 35*(1), 72-78. doi:DOI: 10.1002/phar.1534

Fiatarone, M., O'Neill, E., Ryan, N., Clements, K., Solares, G., Nelson, M., . . . Evans, W. (1994). Exercise Training and Nutritional Supplementation for Physical Frailty in Very Elderly People. *NEJM, 330*(25), 1769-1775. doi:https://doi.org/10.1056/NEJM199406233302501

Finkle, W., Greenland, S., Ridgeway, G., Adams, J., Frasco, M., Cook, M., . . . Hoover, R. (2014). Increased risk of non-fatal myocardial infarction following testosterone therapy prescription in men. *PLoS one, 9*(1). doi:https://doi.org/10.1371/journal.pone.0085805

Fitts, R., Peters, J., Dillon, E., Durham, W., Sheffield-Moore, M., & Urban, R. (2015). Weekly Versus Monthly Testosterone Administration on Fast and Slow Skeletal Muscle Fibers in Older Adult Males. *Journal of Clinical Endocinology and Metabolism, 100*(2), D223-31. doi:https://doi.org/10.1210/jc.2014-2759

Fitts, R., Romatowski, J., Peters, J., Paddon-Jones, D., Wolfe, R., & Ferrando, A. (2007). The deleterious effects of bed rest on human skeletal muscle fibers are exacerbated by hypercortisolemia and ameliorated by dietary supplementation. *American Psychological Society, 293*(1), c313-320. doi:https://doi.org/10.1152/ajpcell.00573.2006

Fleishman, S., Khan, H., Homel, P., Suhail, M., Strebel-Amrhein, R., Mohammad, F., . . . Suppiah, K. (2010). Testosterone levels and quality of life in diverse male patients with cancers unrelated to androgens. *Journal of Clinical Oncology, 28*(34), 5054-60. doi:https://doi.org/10.1200/JCO.2010.30.3818

REFERENCES

Gebel, K., Ding, D., Chey, Stamatakis, E., Brown, W., & Bauman, A. (2015, June). Effect of Moderate to Vigorous Physical Activity on All-Cause Mortality in Middle-aged and Older Australians. *JAMA, 175*(6), 970-7. doi:https://doi.org/10.1001/jamainternmed.2015.0541

Gentil, P., de Lira, C., Paoli, A., Dos Santos, J., da Silva, R., Junior, J., . . . Magosso, R. (2017). Nutrition, Pharmacological and Training Strategies Adopted by Six Bodybuilders: Case Report and Critical Review. *European Journal of Translational Myology, 27*(1), 2647. doi:https://dx.doi.org/10.4081%2Fejtm.2017.6247

Giannoulis, M., Martin, F., Nair, K., Umpleby, A., & Sonksen, P. (2012). Hormone replacement therapy and physical function in healthy older men. Time to talk hormones? *Endocrine Reviews, 33*(3), 314-77. doi:https://doi.org/10.1210/er.2012-1002

Gibney, J., Healy, M., & Sönksen, P. (2007). The Growth Hormone/Insulin-Like Growth Factor-1 Axis in Exercise and Sport. *Endocrine Reviews, 28*(6), 603-624. doi:https://doi.org/10.1210/er.2006-0052

Giordano, R., Bonelli, L., Marinazzo, E., Ghigo, E., & Arvat, E. (2008). Growth hormone treatment in human ageing: benefits and risks. *Hormones, 7*(2), 133-139. Retrieved from http://www.hormones.gr/216/article/article.html

Glaser, R., & Dimitrakakis, C. (2013). Reduced breast cancer incidence in women treated with subcutaneous testosterone, or testosterone with anastrozole: A prospective, observational study. *Maturitas, 76*(4), 342-9. doi:https://doi.org/10.1016/j.maturitas.2013.08.002

Goldstein, I., Stecher, V., & Carlsson, M. (2017). Treatment response to sildenafil in men with erectile dysfunction relative to concomitant comorbidities and age. *International Journal of Clinical Practice, 71*, 3-4. doi:https://doi.org/10.1111/ijcp.12939

Gomez-Cabrera, M., Domenech, E., & Viña, J. (2008, Jan 15). Moderate exercise is an antioxidant: upregulation of antioxidant genes by training. *Free Radical biology and medicine, 44*(2), 126-31. doi:https://doi.org/10.1016/j.freeradbiomed.2007.02.001

Goodman, N., Guay, A., Dandona, P., Dhindsa, S., Faiman, C., & Cunningham, G. (2015). AMERICAN ASSOCIATION OF CLINICAL ENDOCRINOLOGISTS AND AMERICAN COLLEGE OF ENDOCRINOLOGY POSITION STATEMENT ON THE ASSOCIATION OF TESTOSTERONE AND CARDIOVASCULAR RISK. *Endocrine Practice, 21*, 1066-1073. doi:https://doi.org/10.4158/EP14434.PS

Gorgey, A., Khalil, R., Gill, R., O'Brien, L., Lavis, T., Castillo, T., . . . Adler, R. (2017). Effects of Testosterone and Evoked Resistance Exercise after Spinal Cord Injury (TEREX-SCI): study protocol for a randomised controlled trial. *BMJ open, 7*(4). doi:https://doi.org/10.1136/bmjopen-2016-014125

Hackett, G. (2016). Testosterone Replacement Therapy and Mortality in Older Men. *Drug Safety, 39*, 117-130. doi:https://doi.org/10.1007/s40264-015-0348-y

Hackett, G. I., Cole, N. S., Deshpande, A. A., Popple, M. D., Kennedy, D., & Wilkinson, P. (2009). Biochemical hypogonadism in men with type 2 diabetes in primary care practice. *The British Journal of Diabetes & Vascular Disease, 9*(5), 226-31. doi:http://dx.doi.org/10.1177%2F1474651409342635

Haider, A., Yassin, A., Haider, K., Doros, G., Saad, F., & Rosano, G. (2016). Men with testosterone deficiency and a history of cardiovascular diseases benefit from long-term testos-

REFERENCES

terone therapy: observational, real-life data from a registry study. *Health Risk Management, 12,* 251-61. doi:https://doi.org/10.2147/VHRM.S108947

Healthcare Cost and Utilization Project (HCUP). (2014). *HCUP National Inpatient Sample (NIS).* Rockville, MD: Agency for Healthcare Research and Quality. Retrieved from https://www.hcup-us.ahrq.gov/db/nation/nis/tools/stats/NIS_2014_MaskedStats_Core_Weighted.PDF

Högström, G., Nordström, A., & Nordström, P. (2016, Aug). Aerobic fitness in late adolescence and the risk of early death: a prospective cohort study of 1.3 million Swedish men. *International Journal of Epidemeiology, 45*(4), 1159-1168. doi:https://doi.org/10.1093/ije/dyv321

Horstman, A., Dillon, E., Urban, R., & Sheffield-Moore, M. (2012). The Role of Androgens and Estrogens on Healthy Aging and Longevity. *The Journals of Gerentology. Series A, Biological Sciences and Medical Sciences, 67*(11), 1140-1152. doi:https://doi.org/10.1093/gerona/gls068

Hulmi, J., Volek, J., Selänne, H., & Mero, A. (2005). Protein Ingestion Prior to Strength Exercise Affects Blood Hormones and Metabolism. *Medicine and Science in Sports and Exercise, 37*(11), 1990-7. Retrieved from https://www.ncbi.nlm.nih.gov/pubmed/16286871

Huo, S., Scialli, A., McGarvey, S., Hill, E., Tügertimur, B., Hogenmiller, A., . . . Fugh-Berman, A. (2016). Treatment of Men for "Low Testosterone": A Systematic Review. *PLoS one, 11*(9). doi:https://doi.org/10.1371/journal.pone.0162480

Hyde, Z., Flicker, L., Almeida, O., Hankey, G., McCaul, K., Chubb, S., & Yeap, B. (2010). Low free testosterone predicts frailty in older men: the health in men study. *The Journal of*

Clinical Endocrinology and Metabolism, 95(7), 3165-72. doi:https://doi.org/10.1210/jc.2009-2754

Institute of Medicine (US) Committee on Assessing the Need for Clinical Trials. (2004). Testosterone and Aging: Clinical Research Directions. *National Academic Press.*

International Osteoporosis Foundation. (2017). *Facts and Statistics.* Retrieved from International Osteoporosis Foundation: https://www.iofbonehealth.org/facts-statistics

Janssen, H., Samson, M., & Verhaar, H. (2002). Vitamin D deficiency, muscle function, and falls in elderly people. *The American Journal of Clinical Nutrition, 75*(4), 611-5. Retrieved from http://ajcn.nutrition.org/content/75/4/611.long

Jones, T. (2010). Testosterone deficiency: a risk factor for cardiovascular disease? *Trends in Endocrinology and Metabolism, 21*(8), 496-503. doi:https://doi.org/10.1016/j.tem.2010.03.002

Kanayama, G., Hudson, J., DeLuca, J., Isaacs, S., Baggish, A., Weiner, R., . . . Pope, H. J. (2015). Prolonged Hypogonadism in Males Following Withdrawal from Anabolic-Androgenic Steroids: an Underrecognized Problem. *Addictions, 110*(5), 823-831. doi:https://dx.doi.org/10.1111%2Fadd.12850

Khaw, K., Dowsett, M., Folkerd, E., Bingham, S., Wareham, N., Luben, R., . . . Day, N. (2007). Endogenous Testosterone and Mortality Due to All Causes, Cardiovascular Disease, and Cancer in Men. *Circulation, 116,* 2694-2701. doi:https://doi.org/10.1161/CIRCULATIONAHA.107.719005

Kim, J., Oh, S., Shin, J., Hwang, S., Hyun, S., Yang, H., & Lee, G. (2013). Testosterone related good neurologic outcome on the patients with return of spontaneous circulation after cardiac arrest: a prospective cohort study. *Resuscitation,*

REFERENCES

  84(5), 645-50. doi:https://doi.org/10.1016/j.resuscitation.2012.10.022

Kim, S. (2014). Testosterone Replacement Therapy and Bone Mineral Density in Men with Hypogonadism. *Endocrinology and Metabolism, 29*(1), 30-32. doi:https://dx.doi.org/10.3803%2FEnM.2014.29.1.30

Klotzbuecher, C., Ross, P., Landsman, P., Abbott, T. 3., & Berger, M. (2000). Patients with prior fractures have an increased risk of future fractures: a summary of the literature and statistical synthesis. *J Bone Miner Res, 15*(4), 721-39. doi:https://doi.org/10.1359/jbmr.2000.15.4.721

Kovac, J., Rajanahally, S., Smith, R., Coward, R., Lamb, D., & Lipshultz, L. (2014). Patient satisfaction with testosterone replacement therapies: the reasons behind the choices. *Journal of Sexual Medicine, 11*(2), 553-62. doi:https://doi.org/10.1111/jsm.12369

Kraemer, W., & Ratamess, N. (2005). Hormonal Responses and Adaptations to Resistance Exercise and Training. *Sports Medicine, 35*(4), 339-61.

Kraemer, W., Häkkinen, K., Newton, R., Nindl, B., Volek, J., McCormick, M., . . . Evans, W. (1999). Effects of heavy-resistance training on hormonal response patterns in younger vs. older men. *Journal of Applied Physiology, 87*(3), 982-992. Retrieved from http://jap.physiology.org/content/87/3/982.long

Krasnoff, J., Basaria, S., Pencina, M., Jasuja, G., Vasan, R., Ulloor, J., . . . Murabito, J. (2010). Free testosterone levels are associated with mobility limitation and physical performance in community-dwelling men: the Framingham Offspring Study. *The Journal of Clinical Endocrinology and Metabolism, 95*(6), 2790-9. doi:https://doi.org/10.1210/jc.2009-2680

Kvorning, T., Andersen, M., Brixen, K., & Madsen, K. (2006). Suppression of endogenous testosterone production attenuates the response to strength training: a randomized, placebo-controlled, and blinded intervention study. *American Journal of Physiology. Endocrinology and Metabolism, 291*(6), e1325-1332. doi:https://doi.org/10.1152/ajpendo.00143.2006

Laaksonen, D., Niskanen, L., Punnonen, K., Nyyssönen, K., Tuomainen, T., Valkonen, V., . . . Salonen, J. (2004). Testosterone and sex hormone-binding globulin predict the metabolic syndrome and diabetes in middle-aged men. *Diabetes Care, 27*(5), 1036-41. doi:https://doi.org/10.2337/diacare.27.5.1036

Laughlin, G., Barrett-Connor, E., & Bergstrom, J. (2008). Low serum testosterone and mortality in older men. *The Journal of Clinical Endocrinology and Metabolism, 93*(1), 68-75. doi:https://doi.org/10.1210/jc.2007-1792

Laughlin, G., Goodell, V., & Barrett-Connor, E. (2010). Extremes of Endogenous Testosterone Are Associated with Increased Risk of Incident Coronary Events in Older Women. *Journal of Clinical Endocrinology and Metabolism, 95*(2), 740-7. doi:https://doi.org/10.1210/jc.2009-1693

LeBlanc, E., Nielson, C., Marshall, L., Lapidus, J., Barrett-Connor, E., Ensrud, K., . . . Orwoll, E. (2009). The effects of serum testosterone, estradiol, and sex hormone binding globulin levels on fracture risk in older men. *Journal of Clinical Endocrinology and Metabolism, 94*(9), 3337-46. doi:https://doi.org/10.1210/jc.2009-0206

Leder, B., Rohrer, J., Rubin, S., Gallo, J., & Longcope, C. (2004). Effects of Aromatase Inhibition in Elderly Men with Low or Borderline-Low Serum Testosterone Levels. *Journal*

REFERENCES

of Clinical Endocrinology and Metabolism, 89(3), 1174-1180. doi:https://doi.org/10.1210/jc.2003-031467

Li, H., Guo, Y., Yang, Z., Roy, M., & Guo, Q. (2016). The efficacy and safety of oxandrolone treatment for patients with severe burns: A systematic review and meta-analysis. *Burns, 42*(4), 717-27. doi:https://doi.org/10.1016/j.burns.2015.08.023

Liu, H., Bravata, D., Olkin, I., Nayak, S., Roberts, B., Garber, A., & Hoffman, A. (2007). Systematic Review: The Safety and Efficacy of Growth Hormone in the Healthy Elderly. *Annals of Internal Medicine, 146*(2), 104-115. doi:10.7326/0003-4819-146-2-200701160-00005

Longo, V., Antebi, A., Bartke, A., Barzilai, N., Brown-Borg, H. M., Caruso, C., . . . Fontana, L. (2015). Interventions to Slow Aging in Humans: Are We Ready? *Aging cell, 14*(4), 497-510. doi:https://doi.org/10.1111/acel.12338

Maggio, M., Lauretani, F., Ceda, G., Bandinelli, S., Ling, S., Metter, E., . . . Ferrucci, L. (2007). Relationship Between Low Levels of Anabolic Hormones and 6-Year Mortality in Older MenThe Aging in the Chianti Area (InCHIANTI) Study. *Arch Intern Med, 167*(20), 2249-2254. doi:10.1001/archinte.167.20.2249

Maggio, M., Lauretani, F., De Vita, F., Basaria, S., Lippi, G., Butto, V., . . . Ceda, G. (2014). Multiple hormonal dysregulation as determinant of low physical performance and mobility in older persons. *Current Pharmeceutical Design*, 3119-48.

Maggio, M., Nicolini, F., Cattabiani, C., Beghi, C., Gherli, T., Schwartz, R., . . . Ceda, G. (2012). Effects of testosterone supplementation on clinical and rehabilitative outcomes in older men undergoing on-pump CABG. *Contemporary*

Clinical Trials, 33(4), 730-8. doi:https://doi.org/10.1016/j.cct.2012.02.019

Malkin, C., Pugh, P., Morris, P., Asif, S., Jones, T., & Channer, K. (2010). Low serum testosterone and increased mortality in men with coronary heart disease. *Heart, 96*(22), 1821-5. doi:https://doi.org/10.1136/hrt.2010.195412

Malkin, C., Pugh, P., Morris, P., Kerry, K., Jones, R., Jones, T., & Channer, K. (2004). Testosterone replacement in hypogonadal men with angina improves ischemic threshold and quality of life. *Heart, 90*(8), 871-6. doi:https://doi.org/10.1136/hrt.2003.021121

Maradit Kremers, H., Larson, D., Crowson, C., Kremers, W., Washington, R., Steiner, C., . . . Berry, D. (2015). Prevalence of Total Hip and Knee Replacement in the United States. *The Journal of Bone and Joint Surgery. American Volume., 97*(17), 1386-1397. doi:https://doi.org/10.2106/JBJS.N.01141

Mazidi, M., Rezaie, P., Kengne, A., Mobarhan, M., & Ferns, G. (2016, April-June). Gut microbiome and metabolic syndrome. *Diabetes and Metabolic Syndrome: Clinical Research and Reviews, 10*(2 s1), s150-s157. doi:https://doi.org/10.1016/j.dsx.2016.01.024

Mekala, K., & Tritos, N. (2009). Effects of Recombinant Human Growth Hormone Therapy in Obesity in Adults: A Meta-analysis. *Journal of Clinical Endocrinology and Metabolism, 94*(1), 130-137. doi:https://doi.org/10.1210/jc.2008-1357

Menke, A., Guallar, E., Rohrmann, S., Nelson, W., Rifai, N., Kanarek, N., . . . Platz, E. (2010). Sex steroid hormone concentrations and risk of death in US men. *American Journal of Epidemiology, 17*(5), 583-92. doi:https://doi.org/10.1093/aje/kwp415

REFERENCES

Molitch, M., Clemmons, D., Malozowski, S., Merriam, G., & Vance, M. (2011). Evaluation and Treatment of Adult Growth Hormone Deficiency: An Endocrine Society Clinical Practice Guideline. *Journal of Clinical Endocrinology and Metabolism, 96*(6), 1587-1609. doi:https://doi.org/10.1210/jc.2011-0179

Møller, N., & Jørgensen, J. (2009). Effects of Growth Hormone on Glucose, Lipid, and Protein Metabolism in Human Subjects. *Endocrine Reviews, 30*(2), 152-177. doi:https://doi.org/10.1210/er.2008-0027

Morganteler, A. (2015). Testosterone deficiency and cardiovascular mortality. *Asian Journal of Andrology, 17*(1), 26-31. doi:https://dx.doi.org/10.4103%2F1008-682X.143248

Morgentaler, A., Zitzmann, M., Traish, A., Fox, A., Jones, T., Maggi, M., . . . Torres, L. (2016). Fundamental Concepts Regarding Testosterone Deficiency and Treatment: International Expert Consensus Resolutions. *Mayo Clinic Proceedings, 91*(7), 881-96. doi:http://dx.doi.org/10.1016/j.mayocp.2016.04.007

Muniyappa, R., Sorkin, J., Veldhuis, J., Harman, S., Münzer, T., Bhasin, S., & Blackman, M. (2007). Long-term testosterone supplementation augments overnight growth hormone secretion in healthy older men. *American Journal of Physiology. Endocrinology and Metabolism, 293*(3), E769-E775. doi:https://doi.org/10.1152/ajpendo.00709.2006

Muraleedharan, V., Marsh, H., Kapoor, D., Channer, K., & Jones, T. (2013). Testosterone deficiency is associated with increased risk of mortality and testosterone replacement improves survival in men with type 2 diabetes. *European Journal of Endocrinology, 169*(6), 725-33. doi:https://doi.org/10.1530/EJE-13-0321

Myers, J., Kaykha, A., George, S., Abella, J., Zaheer, N., Lear, S., . . . Froelicher, V. (2004, Dec 15). Fitness versus physical activity patterns in predicting mortality in men. *American Journal of Medicine, 117*(12), 912-8. doi:https://doi.org/10.1016/j.amjmed.2004.06.047

Nakamura, K., & Ogata, T. (2016). Locomotive Syndrome: Definition and Management. *Clinical Reviews in Bone and Mineral Metabolism, 14*(2), 56-67. doi:0.1007/s12018-016-9208-2

Nass, R., Park, J., & T. M. (2007). Growth hormone supplementation in the elderly. *Endocrinology and Metabolism clinics of North America, 36*(1), 233-45. doi:https://doi.org/10.1016/j.ecl.2006.08.004

Neto, W., Gama, E., Rocha, L., Ramos, C., Taets, W., Scapini, K., . . . Caperuto, É. (2015). Effects of testosterone on lean mass gain in elderly men: systematic review with meta-analysis of controlled and randomized studies. *Age, 37*(5), 9742. doi:https://doi.org/10.1007/s11357-014-9742-0

Nieschlag, E., & Vorona, E. (2015). MECHANISMS IN ENDOCRINOLOGY: Medical consequences of doping with anabolic androgenic steroids: effects on reproductive functions. *European Journal of Endocrinology, 173*(2), R47-58. doi:https://doi.org/10.1530/EJE-15-0080

Nijs, J., Kosek, E., Van Oosterwijck, J., & Meeus, M. (2012). Dysfunctional endogenous analgesia during exercise in patients with chronic pain: to exercise or not to exercise? *Pain Physician, 15*(3s), e205-213. Retrieved from http://www.painphysicianjournal.com/linkout?issn=1533-3159&vol=15&page=ES205

Oakland, K., Nadler, R., Cresswell, L., Jackson, D., & Coughlin, P. (2016). Systematic review and meta-analysis of the association between frailty and outcome in surgical patients. *Annals of the Royal College of Surgeons of England, 98*(2), 80-85. doi:https://doi.org/10.1308/rcsann.2016.0048

Ohlander, S., Lindgren, M., & Lipshultz, L. (2016). Testosterone and Male Infertility. *The Urologic Clinics of North America, 43*(2), 195-202. doi:https://doi.org/10.1016/j.ucl.2016.01.006

Ohlsson C, B.-C. E., Labrie, F., Karlsson, M., Ljunggren, O., Vandenput, L., Mellström, D., & Tivesten, A. (2011). High serum testosterone is associated with reduced risk of cardiovascular events in elderly men. The MrOS (Osteoporotic Fractures in Men) study in Sweden. *Journal of the American College of Cardiology, 58*(16), 1674-81. doi:https://doi.org/10.1016/j.jacc.2011.07.019

Pederson, B. S. (2006, Feb 1). Evidence for prescribing exercise as therapy in chronic disease. *Scandinavian Journal of Medicine and Science in Sports, 16*(s1), 3–63. doi:10.1111/j.1600-0838.2006.00520.x

Pierpoint, T., McKeigue, P., Isaacs, A., Wild, S., & Jacobs, H. (1998). Mortality of women with polycystic ovary syndrome at long-term follow-up. *Journal of Clinical Epidemiology, 51*(7), 581-6. doi:http://dx.doi.org/10.1016/S0895-4356(98)00035-3

Pope, H. J., & Katz, D. (1994). Psychiatric and Medical effects of anaboli-androgenic steroid use. A controlled study of 160 athletes. *Archives of General Psychiatry, 51*(5), 375-82. doi:doi:10.1001/archpsyc.1994.03950050035004

Pope, H. J., Wood, R., Rogol, A., Nyberg, F., Bowers, L., & Bhasin, S. (2014, 2014). Adverse Health Consequences of Performance-Enhancing Drugs: An Endocrine Society

Scientific Statement. *Endocrinology Review, 35*(3), 341-75. doi:https://doi.org/10.1210/er.2013-1058

Puggaard, L. (2005). Age-Related Decline in Maximal Oxygen Capacity: Consequences for Performance of Everyday Activities. *Journal of the American Geriatrics Society, 53*(3), 546-7. doi:https://doi.org/10.1111/j.1532-5415.2005.53178_3.x

Rahnema, C., Crosnoe, L., & Kim, E. (2015). Designer steroids - over-the-counter supplements and their androgenic component: review of an increasing problem. *Andrology, 3*(2), 150-155. doi:https://doi.org/10.1111/andr.307

Randeva, H., Tan, B., Weickert, M., Lois, K., Nestler, J., Sattar, N., & Lehnert, H. (2012). Cardiometabolic Aspects of the Polycystic Ovary Syndrome. *Endocrine Review, 33*(5), 812-841. doi:https://doi.org/10.1210/er.2012-1003

Rasmussen, J., Selmer, C., Østergren, P., Pedersen, K., Schou, M., Gustafsson, F., . . . Kistorp, C. (2016). Former Abusers of Anabolic Androgenic Steroids Exhibit Decreased Testosterone levels and Hypogonadal Symptoms Years after Cessation: A Case-Control Study. *PLoS One, 11*(8). doi:https://doi.org/10.1371/journal.pone.0161208

Regis, L., Celma, A., Planas, J., deTorres, I., Ferrer, R., & Morote, J. (2015). Determined Free Serum Testosterone is Better than Total Testosterone as a Predictor of Prostate Cancer Risk. *International Journal of Research Studies in Biosciences, 3*(9), 22-32. Retrieved from https://www.google.com/url?sa=t&rct=j&q=&esrc=s&source=web&cd=1&cad=rja&uact=8&ved=0ahUKEwiGw7a1zZXUAhWCPCYKHdo_ADwQFggtMAA&url=https%3A%2F%2Fwww.arcjournals.org%2Fpdfs%2Fijrsb%2Fv3-i9%2F4.

REFERENCES

pdf&usg=AFQjCNHkA-NQf7uq42uokLL_340FycPeyA&sig2=Thr5berq4S3kOJAc3v

Ross, R., Hill, J., Latimer, A., & Day, A. (2016, Mar). Evaluating a small change approach to preventing long term weight gain in overweight and obese adults--Study rationale, design, and methods. *Contemporary Clinical Trials, 47*, 275-81. doi:https://doi.org/10.1016/j.cct.2016.02.001

Rossow, L., Fukuda, D., Fahs, C., Loenneke, J., & Stout, J. (2013). Natural bodybuilding competition preparation and recovery: a 12-month case study. *International Journal of Sports Physiology and Performance, 8*(5), 582-92. doi:10.1123/ijspp.8.5.582

Roy, C., Snyder, P., Stephens-Shields, A., Artz, A., Bhasin, S., Cohen, H., . . . Ellenberg, S. S. (2017). Association of Testosterone Levels With Anemia in Older Men: A Controlled Clinical Trial. *JAMA Internal Medicine, 177*(4), 480-490. doi:https://doi.org/10.1001/jamainternmed.2016.9540

Rudman, D., Feller, A., Nagraj, H., Gergans, G., Lalitha, P., Goldberg, A., . . . Mattson, D. (1990). Effects of Human Growth Hormone in Men Over 60 Years Old. *New England Journal of Medicine, 323*(1), 1-6. doi:https://doi.org/10.1056/NEJM199007053230101

Saad F, Y. A. (2016). Effects of long-term treatment with testosterone on weight and waist size in 411 hypogonadal men with obesity classes I-III: observational data from two registry studies. *International Journal of Obesity, 40*(1), 162-70. doi:https://doi.org/10.1038/ijo.2015.139

Saad, F., Yassin, A., Haider, A., Doros, G., & Gooren, L. (2015). Elderly men over 65 years of age with late-onset hypogonadism benefit as much from testosterone treatment as do younger men. *Korean Journal of Urology, 56*, 310-317. doi:https://doi.org/10.4111/kju.2015.56.4.310

Samaras, N., Papadopoulou, M., Samaras, D., & Ongaro, F. (2014). Off-label use of hormones as an antiaging strategy: a review. *Clinical Interventions in Aging, 9*, 1175-1186. doi:https://dx.doi.org/10.2147%2FCIA.S48918

Samaras, N., Samaras, D., Lang, P., Forster, A., Pichard, C., Frangos, E., & Meyer, P. (2013). A view of geriatrics through hormones. What is the relation between andropause and well-known geriatric syndromes? *Maturitas, 74*(3), 213-9. doi:https://doi.org/10.1016/j.maturitas.2012.11.009

Sanchis-Gomar, F., Olaso-Gonzalez, G., Corella, D., Gomez-Cabrera, M., & Vina, J. (2011, Aug). Increased average longevity among the "Tour de France" cyclists. *International journal of sports medicine, 32*(8), 644-7. doi:https://doi.org/10.1055/s-0031-1271711

Santos, M., Sayegh, A., Groehs, R., Fonseca, G., Trombetta, I., Barretto, A., . . . Alves, M. (2015). Testosterone Deficiency Increases Hospital Readmission and Mortality Rates in Male Patients with Heart Failure. *Arquivos Brasileiros Cardiologia, 105*(3), 256–264. doi:https://dx.doi.org/10.5935%2Fabc.20150078

Sattler, F., Bhasin, S., He, J., Yarasheski, K., Binder, E., Schroeder, E., . . . Azen, S. (2011). Durability of the effects of testosterone and growth hormone supplementation in older community dwelling men: the HORMA trial. *Clinical Endocrinology, 75*(1), 103-111. doi:https://doi.org/10.1111/j.1365-2265.2011.04014.x

Scovell, J., Ramasamy, R., & Kovac, J. (2014). A critical analysis of testosterone supplementation therapy and cardiovascular

REFERENCES

risk in elderly men. *Canadian Urological Association Journal, 8*(5-6). doi:http://dx.doi.org/10.5489/cuaj.1962

Sheffield-Moore, M., Dillon, E., Casperson, S., Gilkison, C., Paddon-Jones, D., Durham, W., . . . Urban, R. (2011). A Randomized Pilot Study of Monthly Cycled Testosterone Replacement or Continuous Testosterone Replacement Versus Placebo in Older Men. *Journal of Clinical Endocrinology and Metabolism, 96*(11), E1831-1837. doi:https://doi.org/10.1210/jc.2011-1262

Shephard, R., & Futcher, R. (1997). Physical activity and cancer: how may protection be maximized. *Critical Reviews in Oncogenesis, 8*(2-3), 219-72. Retrieved from https://www.ncbi.nlm.nih.gov/pubmed/9570295

Shin, Y., You, J., Cha, J., & Park, J. (2016). The relationship between serum total testosterone and free testosterone levels with serum hemoglobin and hematocrit levels: a study in 1221 men. *Aging Male, 19*(4), 209-214. doi:https://doi.org/10.1080/13685538.2016.1229764

Shores, M., Arnold, A., Biggs, M., Longstreth, W. J., Smith, N., Kizer, J., . . . Matsumoto, A. (2014). Testosterone and Dihydrotestosterone and Incident Ischemic Stroke in Men in the Cardiovascular Health Study. *Clinical Endocrinology, 81*(5), 746-753. doi:https://doi.org/10.1111/cen.12452

Shores, M., Biggs, M., Arnold, A., Smith, N., Longstreth, W. J., Kizer, J., . . . Matsumoto, A. (2014). Testosterone, Dihydrotestosterone, and Incident Cardiovascular Disease and Mortality in the Cardiovascular Health Study. *Journal of Clinical Endocrinology and Metabolism, 99*(6), 2061-2068. doi:https://dx.doi.org/10.1210%2Fjc.2013-3576

Sievers, C., Klotsche, J., Pieper, L., Schneider, H., März, W., Wittchen, H., . . . Mantzoros, C. (2010). Low testosterone levels predict all-causes mortality and cardiovascular events in women: a prospective cohort study in German primary care patients. *European Journal of Endocrinology, 163*(4), 699-708. doi:https://doi.org/10.1530/EJE-10-0307

Snyder, G., & Shoskes, D. (2016). Hypogonadism and testosterone replacement therapy in end-stage renal disease (ESRD) and transplant patients. *Translational Andrology and Urology, 5*(6), 885-889. doi:https://dx.doi.org/10.21037%2Ftau.2016.08.01

Snyder, P. (2004). Hypogonadism in Elderly Men- What to Do Until the Evidence Comes. *New England Journal of Medicine, 350*(5), 440-2. doi:https://doi.org/10.1056/NEJMp038207

Spitzer, M., Huang, G., Basaria, S., Travison, T., & Bhasin, S. (2013). Risk and benefits of testosterone therapy in older men. *Nature Reviews. Endocrinology, 9*(7), 414-24. doi:https://doi.org/10.1038/nrendo.2013.73

Srinivas-Shankar, U., Roberts, S., Connolly, M., O'Connell, M., Adams, J., Oldham, J., & Wu, F. (2010). Effects of Testosterone on Muscle Strength, Physical Function, Body Composition, and Quality of Life in Intermediate-Frail Elderly Men: A Randomized, Double-Blind, Placebo-Controlled Study. *Clinical Endocrinology and Metabolism, 95*(2), 639-650. doi:https://doi.org/10.1210/jc.2009-1251

Stergiopoulos, K., Brennan, J., Mathews, R., Setaro, J., & Kort, S. (2008). Anabolic steroids, acute myocardial infarction and polycythemia: A case report and review of the literature. *Vascular Health Risk Management, 4*(6), 1475-1480.

REFERENCES

Retrieved from https://www.ncbi.nlm.nih.gov/pmc/articles/PMC2663437/?report=reader#__ffn_sectitle

Tang, W., & Hazen, S. (2014, Oct 1). The contributory role of gut microbiota in cardiovascular disease. *The Journal of Clinical Investigation, 124*(10), 4204–4211. doi:https://dx.doi.org/10.1172%2FJCI72331

Thompson, P., Franklin, B., Balady, G., Blair, S., Corrado, D., Estes, N. 3., . . . Costa, F. (2007, May 1). Exercise and acute cardiovascular events placing the risks into perspective: a scientific statement from the American Heart Association Council on Nutrition, Physical Activity, and Metabolism and the Council on Clinical Cardiology. *Circulation, 115*(17), 2358-68. doi:https://doi.org/10.1161/CIRCULATIONAHA.107.181485

Tracz, M., Sideras, K., Boloña, E., Haddad, R., Kennedy, C., Uraga, M., . . . Montori, V. (2006). Clinical Review: Testosterone Use in Men and Its Effects on Bone Health. A Systematic Review and Meta-analysis of Randomized Placebo-Controlled Trials. *The Journal of Clinical Endocrinology and Metabolism, 9*(16), 2011-2016. doi:https://doi.org/10.1210/jc.2006-0036

Travison, T., Basaria, S., Storer, T., Jette, A., Miciek, R., Farwell, W., . . . Brooks, B. (2011). Clinical Meaningfulness of the Changes in Muscle Performance and Physical and Function Associated with Testosterone Administration In Older Men With Mobility Limitation. *J Gerontol A Biol Sci Med Sci, 66*(10), 1090-99. doi:https://doi.org/10.1093/gerona/glr100

Travison, T., Morley, J., Araujo, A., O'Donnel, I. A., & McKinlay, J. (2006). The Relationship between Libido and Testosterone Levels in Aging Men. *The Journal of Clinical Endo-*

crinology and Metabolism, 91(7), 2509-2513. doi:https://doi.org/10.1210/jc.2005-2508

Tricker, R., Casaburi, R., Storer, T., Clevenger, B., Berman, N., Shirazi, A., & Bhasin, S. (1996). The effects of supra-physiological doses of testosterone on angry behavior in healthy eugonadal men-a clinical research center study. *Journa of Clinical Endocrinology and Metabolism, 81*(10), 3754-8. doi:https://doi.org/10.1210/jcem.81.10.8855834

Vandenput, L., Mellström, D., Laughlin, G., Cawthon, P., Cauley, J., Hoffman, A., . . . Ohlsson, C. (2017). Low Testosterone, but Not Estradiol, Is Associated With Incident Falls in Older Men: The International MrOS Study. *Journal of Bone and Mineral Research.* doi:https://doi.org/10.1002/jbmr.3088

Vermeulen, A., & Verdonck, G. (1992). Representativeness of a single point plasma testosterone level for the long term hormonal milieu in men. *Journal of Clinical Endocrinology and Metabolism, 74*(4), 939-42. doi:https://doi.org/10.1210/jcem.74.4.1548361

Vigen, R., O'Donnell, C., Barón, A., Grunwald, G., Maddox, T., Bradley, S., . . . Ho, P. (2013). Association of testosterone therapy with mortality, myocardial infarction, and stroke in men with low testosterone levels. *JAMA, 310*(17), 1829-36. doi:https://doi.org/10.1001/jama.2013.280386

Vina, J., Sanchis-Gomar, F., Martinez-Bello, V., & Gomez-Cabrera, M. (2012, September). Exercise acts as a drug; the pharmacological benefits of exercise. *British Journal of Pharmacology, 167*(1), 1-12. doi:https://dx.doi.org/10.1111%2Fj.1476-5381.2012.01970.x

Vitale, G., Cesari, M., & Mari, D. (2016). Aging of the endocrine system and its potential impact on sarcopenia. *European*

REFERENCES

Journal of Internal Medicine, 35, 10-15. doi:https://doi.org/10.1016/j.ejim.2016.07.017

Warburton, D., Nicol, C., & Bredin, S. (2006, Mar 14). Health benefits of physical activity: the evidence. *Canadian Medical Association Journal, 174*(6), 801-809. doi:https://dx.doi.org/10.1503%2Fcmaj.051351

Weissberger, A., Anastasiadis, A., Sturgess, I., Martin, F., Smith, M., & Sönksen, P. (2003). Recombinant human growth hormone treatment in elderly patients undergoing elective total hip replacement. *Clinical Endocrinology, 58*(1), 99-107. doi:10.1046/j.1365-2265.2003.01700.x

Wen, C., Wai, J., Tsai, M., Yang, Y., Cheng, T., Lee, M., . . . Wu, X. (2011, Oct 1). Minimum amount of physical activity for reduced mortality and extended life expectancy: a prospective cohort study. *Lancet, 378*(9798), 1244-53. doi:http://dx.doi.org/10.1016/S0140-6736(11)60749-6

Westerman, M., Charchenko, C., Ziegelmann, M., Bailey, G., Nippoldt, T., & Trost, L. (2016). Heavy Testosterone Use Among Bodybuilders: An Uncommon Cohort of Illicit Substance Users. *Mayo Clinic Proceedings, 91*(2), 175-182. doi:https://doi.org/10.1016/j.mayocp.2015.10.027

Wierman, M., Arlt, W., Basson, R., Davis, S., Miller, K., Murad, M., . . . Santoro, N. (2014). Androgen therapy in women: a reappraisal: an Endocrine Society clinical practice guideline. *Journal of Clinical Endocrinology and Metabolism, 99*(10), 3489-510. doi:https://doi.org/10.1210/jc.2014-2260

Wild, S., Pierpoint, T., McKeigue, P., & Jacobs, H. (2000). Cardiovascular disease in women with polycystic ovary syndrome at long-term follow-up: a retrospective cohort study. *Clinical Endocrinology, 52*(5), 595-600. doi:10.1046/j.1365-2265.2000.01000.x

Willoughby, D., Spillane, M., & Schwarz, N. (2014). Heavy Resistance Training and Supplementation with the Alleged Testosterone Booster NMDA Has No Effect on Body Composition, Muscle Performance, and Serum Hormones Associated with the Hypothalamus-Pituitary-Gonadal Axis in Resistance-Trained Males. *Journal of Sports Science and Medicine, 13*(1), 192-199. Retrieved from https://www.ncbi.nlm.nih.gov/pmc/articles/PMC3918557/

Woolston, C. (2011, September 12). The Healthy Skeptic: Products make testosterone claims. *Los Angeles Times.* Retrieved from http://articles.latimes.com/2011/sep/12/health/la-he-skeptic-testosterone-supplements-20110912

Xu, L., Freeman, G., Cowling, B., & Schooling, C. (2013). Testosterone therapy and cardiovascular events among men. A systematic review and meta-analysis of placebo-controlled randomized trials. *BMC Medicine, 11*(108). doi:https://doi.org/10.1186/1741-7015-11-108

Yassin DJ, Y. A. (2014). Combined testosterone and vardenafil treatment for restoring erectile function in hypogonadal patients who failed to respond to testosterone therapy alone. *Journal of Sexual Medicine, 11*(2), 543-52. doi:https://doi.org/10.1111/jsm.12378

Yeap, B., Alfonso, H., Chubb, S., Hankey, G., Handelsman, D., Golledge, J., . . . Norman, P. (2014). In older men, higher plasma testosterone or dihydrotestosterone are independent predictors for reduced incidence of stroke but not myocardial infarction. *Journal of Clinical Endocrinology and Metabolism, 99*(12), 4565-4573. doi:https://doi.org/10.1210/jc.2014-2664

Zhang, L., Shin, Y., Kim, J., & Park, J. (2016). Could Testosterone Replacement Therapy in Hypogonadal Men Ameliorate

REFERENCES

Anemia, a Cardiovascular Risk Factor? An Observational, 54-Week Cumulative Registry Study. *The Journal of Urology, 195*(4), 1057-64. doi:https://doi.org/10.1016/j.juro.2015.10.130

Zheng, Y., Shen, X., Zhou, Y., Ma, J., Shang, X., & Shi, y. (2015). Effect and safety of testosterone undecanoate in the treatment of late-onset hypogonadism: a meta-analysis. *PubMed Journals, 21*(3), 263-271. Retrieved from https://www.ncbi.nlm.nih.gov/labs/articles/25898560/

Made in the USA
Lexington, KY
13 July 2017